First Do No Harm:
Clinical Negligence Basics

Dr David Holding
MA, PhD, LLM, Dip Law, PGCEd

First published in Great Britain in 2023 by
Words are Life
10 Chester Place,
Adlington, Chorley, PR6 9RP
wordsarelife@mail.com
www.wordsarelife.co.uk

Electronic version and paperback versions available for purchase on Amazon.
Copyright (c) Dr David Holding and Words are Life.

First edition 2023.

The right of Dr David Holding to be identified as the author of this work has been asserted by him in accordance with the Copyright, Design and Patents Act 1988.

All rights reserved. Without limiting the rights under copyright reserved above, no part of this publication may be reproduced, stored or introduced into a retrieval system, or transmitted, in any form or by any means (electronic, mechanical, photocopying, recording or otherwise), without the prior written permission of both the copyright owner and the publisher of this book. No paragraph of this publication may be reproduced, copied or transmitted save with written permission or in accordance with the provisions of the Copyright Act 1956 (as amended).

ABOUT THE AUTHOR

Dr David Holding studied history at Manchester University before entering the teaching profession in the 1970s. He taught in both state and independent sectors. During this time, he continued historical research culminating in both a Master's degree and a Doctorate. Having previously studied law, David gained a Master of Law degree in Medical Law, which enabled him to transfer to teaching legal courses at university. Since retiring, David has concentrated his research and writing on various aspects of local history, legal trials, forensic science and medico-legal topics.

ALSO BY DAVID HOLDING

Murder in the Heather: The Winter Hill Murder of 1838

This book is a unique account of a brutal murder that occurred on the summit of Winter Hill in Lancashire in 1838. The account draws on both contemporary media reports and court transcripts and examines the events leading to the killing of a 21-year-old packman. It details the trial proceedings of the only suspect in the case. The work concludes with a re-assessment of the case in the light of modern forensic investigation. The reader is invited to reach their own 'verdict' based on the evidence provided.

The Pendle Witch Trials of 1612

The book provides readers with a sequential overview of the famous chain of events that ultimately led to the execution of women accused of practising witchcraft in the county of Lancashire. It is presented as a chronological account of the famous trials at Lancaster Castle in 1612. This book introduces the evidence and interview transcripts that formed the major plank of the prosecution case and will appeal to both the general reader and local historian.

The Dark Figure: Crime in Victorian Bolton

This book provides an absorbing overview of crime in the

Lancashire town of Bolton over the period 1850 to 1890. It is primarily based on documentary survey and analysis of court and police records covering the period. It assesses changes in crime over time and asks whether these relate to economic, social or political changes taking place at the same time. The reader is left to reflect on whether crime (in all its many forms) has changed over time.

Bleak Christmas: The Pretoria Colliery Disaster Of 1910

This work charts the events of the Lancashire Pretoria Pit disaster in December 1910. It reflects on the devastation it left to many local communities whose main source of employment was coal. The main sources analysed are the Home Office Report on the disaster and the Report of the Inquest. The findings of these detailed legal reports are presented in a format that will supplement existing material on the event. The book will also provide a reference source both for local historians and the interested general reader.

Doctors in The Dock: The Trials of Doctors Harold Shipman, John Bodkin Adams and Buck Ruxton

This book takes the reader on a journey into the world of three medical doctors in England, each coming from a different social background but with one common thread going through their lives. They all stood trial for murder. In each case, the reader is presented with all relevant evidence available to jurors in the case. The overall aim of this work is to invite readers to exercise their judgment in reaching a verdict.

The three books within this collection are also available individually:

The Last Temptation: The Trial of Dr Harold Shipman.

The Trial of Dr Buck Ruxton.

The Trial of Dr John Bodkin Adams.

Forensic Science Basics: Every Contact Leaves a Trace

This work is an absorbing introductory study of the techniques familiar from numerous trials, media reports and TV crime dramas. It begins with the basic principles of forensic science and then examines such aspects as the time of death, causes of death, weapons of crime, identification of offenders and much more. It provides essential reading for those who wish to gain a basic introduction to this fascinating area of science.

A Warning from History: The Influenza Pandemic Of 1918

The 1918 Influenza Pandemic was one of the most deadly events in human history, and understanding the events and experience of 1918 is of great importance to pandemic preparation. This book aims to address questions concerning the pandemic's origin, features and causes to provide the reader with an appreciation of the 1918 pandemic and its implications for future pandemics. This work caters to both the science-orientated and general reader in this crucial area of global and public health.

The Lady Chatterley Trial Revisited

The 1960 obscenity trial of Lady Chatterley's Lover remains a symbol of freedom of expression. It is also a seminal case in British literary and social history and is credited as the catalyst which encouraged frank discussion of sexual behaviour. This book introduces readers to the trial itself, describing the prosecution and defence opening and closing speeches to the jury and much more before culminating in the judge's summing-up and the final verdict. The reader is provided with all the evidence to reach a considered assessment of the case and a question to consider. Can certain literature 'actually' corrupt, or does it simply encourage expensive court trials and boost sales?

The Oscar Wilde Trials Revisited

It is only given to very few people to be the principal figure in three Old Bailey trials, before three different judges, and at three consecutive court sessions, all in one year. This complexity is one of the fascinations of the 1895 Oscar Wilde trials. In addition, they embodied celebrity, sex, humorous dialogue, outstanding displays of advocacy and political intrigue woven with issues of art and morality. Wilde's prosecution of the Marquess of Queensberry for criminal libel, and Wilde's later prosecution for 'gross indecency', reveal a complex person at odds with a class-centred and morally ambiguous Victorian society. This work considers these famous trials in chronological sequence and invites the reader to participate as an observer and potential juror in the proceedings. Finally, the reader is encouraged to consider the evidence presented at each trial and arrive at their own conclusions. This work will be of particular interest to law students owing to the counsel's skilfully demonstrated advocacy skills. It also caters for the general reader with a particular interest in presenting criminal cases in the courts in England.

The Whitechapel Murders of 1888

The killing of five women in the Whitechapel area of East London in 1888 remains the greatest and most horrendous of all unsolved murder mysteries. It is the classic cold case. This work takes a novel look into the case from the perspective of the criminal investigation itself. In this approach, the more speculative and conspiratorial theories surrounding the 'Jack the Ripper' crimes have been avoided. The reader is offered insights into these murders by employing the modern forensic techniques of geographical and offender profiling, which shed new light on these serial killings.

Forensic Pathology Basics: The Dead Do Tell a Story

In this work, the reader is taken on a sequential journey of discovery into the fascinating world of forensic pathology, with no previous knowledge of the subject being required of readers. Beginning with the initial discovery of a body, the reader experiences the processes involving the forensic pathologist from the initial examination and identification of the deceased to the final autopsy. The reader will be introduced to practical applications of the pathologist's skills and techniques at each stage. Past criminal cases will be introduced to demonstrate the variety of scenarios in which the assistance of the forensic pathologist is vital. The overall aim of this work is to provide the reader with a fascinating insight into the largely unseen involvement of the forensic pathologist in death investigations. It is especially fascinating when the circumstances involve criminal activity. The manner and causes of death are discussed in detail and cover the main areas of injury. A glossary of medical terminology is provided to explain the various terms used in the text. The work concludes with a selected bibliography to enable the reader to pursue their research in those areas they find particularly interesting and relevant.

The Coronavirus Pandemic: An English Perspective

The Coronavirus (COVID-19) pandemic of 2020 onwards has been described as the second most deadly event in recent human history. The first was attributed to the influenza pandemic of 1918. A comparison has been made between the two events because of the similarities regarding high mortality and because of the resultant impact the pandemics had on the social and economic structures of the countries involved. This work provides the reader with a comprehensive background to the virus's origins, its subsequent rapid spread in England, and the government's responses and control policies implemented to halt its progress. This work will be of interest to both the science-orientated and the general reader with concern in this vital area of public health and in the preparation for future pandemics.

Live Or Let Die? The Euthanasia Debate Revisited

Euthanasia is concerned with decisions relating to the 'end of life', and is a major focus for public, academic and legal debate. Emotional responses dominate and range from calls for more liberalisation to dire warnings that society has now embarked upon a 'slippery slope'. The legal and ethical issues which flow from the euthanasia debate encompass a wide range of matters which permeate medical law by questioning the respective roles of both the medical and legal professions. This work considers definitions of euthanasia, case studies and related law in the UK and Netherlands. This work emphasises the powerful struggle that exists in law, medicine and ethics regarding the nature, scope and foundations of the right to choose the manner of one's own death. Our thought-provoking conclusion considers: "Under what conditions, if any, is it permissible for patients and health professionals to intentionally end life?"

The Psychological Aspects of Eyewitness Evidence

Eyewitness evidence is typically given the most credibility in courts of law. However, it should be admitted with caution and a clear understanding that certain psychological factors can its reliability. This work invites the reader to consider these factors. Each chapter in the work considers the various stages involved in eyewitness testimony in courts of law, from the initial witnessing of an event, the questioning stage and culminating in the court trial itself, and the evidence's presentation. This work poses two questions for the reader to consider: "Exactly how reliable is eyewitness testimony?" and "What factors impact the accuracy of such evidence?"

Justice Delayed: Hillsborough Revisited

This work provides details of the official inquiries launched, post-Hillsborough, together with the new inquests and the criminal trials after. It is also an account of how the British establishment failed to deliver justice at every level and records a catalogue of failings in response to this major disaster. A 'grand scale' conspiracy went right to the top of the establishment and persisted because of collusion between the 'elites' in politics, police and media. But... the Hillsborough families prevailed against all the odds and retained their dignity in the face of great adversity. The reader is left to consider one vital question. "How did Parliament allow such injustice on this scale to remain for so long? The lasting lesson from this disaster is that there must never again, be any arbitrary time limit on justice and accountability.

Beyond Reasonable Doubt: The Jenkins Case Revisited

Most people will have heard of the murder of 13-year-old, Billie-Jo Jenkins in February 1997, in Hastings, East Sussex, and the discovery of her body by her foster father, Sion Jenkins. Everyone will have their own views as to what happened on that fateful day. This raises two pertinent questions. Where do we get our views from? And, what makes us think that we can possibly have any idea as to what actually happened? The chief suspect, Billie-Jo's foster father, Sion Jenkins, was subjected to a 'lynch mob' mentality, largely fuelled by the media and to seemingly endless legal processes. It became increasingly obvious that the police and some members of the judiciary, together with people that Jenkins considered friends (including his ex-wife) had a large part to play in what became a nightmare which Jenkins had to endure. This lasted from the day he discovered the body of Billie-Jo until he was finally acquitted, after having faced six years in prison, two appeals, and three criminal trials. This work exposes the deep failing of the criminal justice system. The deliberate tainting of the Jenkins children's evidence by the police, the failure by the police and CPS to disclose relevant information, together with attempts by the police at putting ideas into the head at Lois, Jenkins' ex-wife. Most people have faith in the criminal justice system, hence the saying 'mud sticks', because they cannot imagine that it can get it so wrong. Yet, the criminal justice system is damaged as is clearly demonstrated in this work. In this work, the reader is presented with the opportunity of experiencing a case which has become one of the greatest 'causes celebre' in British criminal history. The reader is invited to consider their own verdict based upon all the evidence presented to the juries in the three criminal trials. In arriving at their own conclusions, the reader will be able to balance the effects of ineptitude, confirmation bias, media 'hype', innuendo and misinformation, all of which were in plentiful supply in this case. This book brings into sharp focus the fact that it is unquestionably preferred to have all guilty people walk free than to have one innocent person in prison. At the heart of this case lies the truism that as soon as assumptions are made which are not supported by evidence, then the defendant in any criminal case faces an uphill struggle to obtain justice. Guilt must always be proven 'Beyond Reasonable Doubt'.

The Ukrainian Conflict: A British Perspective. Book One – The Year 2022

The Russian invasion of Ukraine in February 2022 is regarded as the greatest threat to the peace and security of Europe since the end of the Cold War. The objective of this work is to provide readers with an overview and assessment of the current conflict in Ukraine. To ensure a 'balanced' perspective, this work draws particular attention to the social, political, economic and military aspects of the war. The reader is presented with an analysis of the conflict on a month-by-month account based upon both media reporting and intelligence releases in both the US and the UK. The work commences with the initial invasion and progresses to the end of year 2022. Included in the work is a selection of 'Commentaries' written by military and political observers of the present Ukrainian conflict based on their own experiences. These are both personal and thought-provoking reflections. Their inclusion will provide the reader with an overview of the conflict and inform on the implications of the war for both the present and foreseeable future.

"Primum
non
nocere"

"First Do No Harm"

Hippocrates of Cos (c 460-377 BC)

In Memoriam

This work is dedicated to the late fellow academic historian, researcher and my loyal friend, Dr John F Henry, in gratitude for his unfailing support, encouragement and wise counsel, so generously extended to me over years of study and research together.

John Felice Henry, 1929-2023

Acknowledgements

I am most grateful for the generous support and encouragement I have received from numerous sources during the course of my research. In particular, I thank members of both the medical and legal professions for the benefit of their opinions on the issues raised in this work. My appreciation also extends to the law staff at the Universities of Manchester and Central Lancashire for their valuable suggestions and observations. I must also include the numerous staff at the various resource centres, archives and libraries I have consulted during the course of my research. My gratitude loses no sincerity in its generality.

Finally, but never least, my gratitude and thanks must always extend to my ever-supportive publisher and valued friend, Lesley Atherton. It is Lesley who provides me with that vital incentive to drive me ever forward in my continued research.

David Holding, 2023

Contents

Introduction

The basic core of medical law is centred upon the dynamic of the doctor-patient relationship. The key to an understanding and analysis of medical law generally, and 'clinical negligence' in particular, is to consider whether the decisions concerning medical practice should lie with doctors themselves, or whether patients have the right to control the decision-making process.

Of particular significance in this respect is the question of whether the medical profession itself, rather than the law, should remain the sole judge of its own profession and membership, with regard to allegations of clinical negligence. Attention is drawn to the fact that there are already in place in the UK a number of quasi-judicial bodies which have been established to oversee aspects of medical practice. However, it is also significant that medical legislation itself has expanded considerably over the past decade, together with the interpretation placed upon it by the courts. It is particularly emphasised within medical law that consent to medical treatment remains a vital element, particularly when doctors have to intervene in situations of emergency treatment.

This work will focus upon the everyday issues of the role of the law in relation to medical practice, and the doctor-patient relationship. Readers are introduced to the nature of legal actions brought by patients against doctors and health care professionals, for damages to compensate them for injuries caused to them. Such injuries may arise out of treatment undertaken by a patient, or it may be that a patient's illness was not diagnosed adequately and was, as a result, left untreated.

The reader's attention is particularly drawn to the three basic elements comprising the 'tort of negligence'. These are, duty of care, breach of that duty and causation.

In general terms, duty of care is an undertaking by a doctor towards his or her patient, to 'exercise the skill and care of a reasonable professional'.

Negligence refers to the failure to reach that standard, thus constituting the breach of duty.

Causation is the legal concept by which a defendant in a legal action is held responsible for his or her conduct, resulting in injury or harm to a patient. The law requires that the doctor's negligent acts or omission to act, constitute a detrimental difference to the patient's well-being. This is referred to in actions for negligence, as the 'but for' principle. Simply put, this means that, 'but for' the actions of the defendant, the patient would have avoided the injury or harm which resulted.

Litigation between patients and doctors has long been recognised as an unsatisfactory means of regulating the doctor/patient relationship. However, the system of tort litigation still remains the principal process by which patients are compensated for their harm within the UK's current legal system.

The perceived difficulties inherent in the tort system, is that it is expensive, there are undue delays between injury and compensation, and such litigation has a disproportionate impact on the National Health Service in the UK. It was only in the late 1990s that a review was commissioned into the Civil Justice System. This was undertaken by a senior British judge, Lord Woolf, who published his final report, *Access to Justice* in 1996.

In it, the judge set out a number of enlightened and progressive objectives by which the civil justice system can be administered more effectively, and which would form the basis for change.

This work is intended to appeal to a wide range of readers including law and medical students seeking a brief introduction to the law in regard to medical practice in the UK. It will also appeal to the lay reader, as a brief guide to issues regarding litigation, and also to ongoing debates surrounding the more questionable and sometimes emotive aspects of everyday medical practice.

The work commences by introducing readers to the definitions of negligence in general, and clinical negligence in particular. This is followed by a brief description of the origins and development of the National Health Service in the UK, which charts its growth and expansion from the 1940s to the present day. The third chapter provides the reader with a general introduction to the basic principles of clinical negligence, while chapter four centres upon the issues of autonomy and consent to medical treatment. The fifth chapter provides a step-by-step examination of the process of clinical negligence litigation, drawing particular attention to the strict rules inherent in entering into litigation. In the final chapter, readers are presented with three case studies, each highlighting a particular aspect of clinical negligence which has been presented in this work, and how these progress through the court system.

A bibliography and reference section has also been included to enable readers to continue their own research into those aspects they find particular relevant to their own studies or which are of particular general interest.

CHAPTER ONE

Definitions

Etymologically, the word tort comes from the legal-French signifying any wrong, which itself is derived from the Latin word 'tortum' meaning twisted. Tort is essentially a civil wrong, as opposed to a crime which is a violation of statutory law. The tort of nis a legal wrong that is suffered by someone at the hands of another who fails to take proper care to avoid what a reasonable person would regard as a foreseeable risk. In many cases there will be a contractual relationship between the parties involved, such as a doctor and patient, employer and employee.

The civil law relating to negligence has evolved and expanded to deal with situations that arise between two or more parties, even where there is no contractual relationship, either written or implied between them.

The case often quoted as the foundation of the current law on negligence is that of Donaghue v Stevenson (1932) AC 562. It was held that, despite there being no contract (express or implied) an action for negligence could succeed. The claimant (plaintiff) in this case successfully argued that she was entitled to a duty of care even though the deficient goods (a bottle of ginger beer with a snail in it) was bought not by herself but by a friend, so that no direct contract existed between the manufacturer of the goods and the person suffering the damage. From this case evolved the principle that we each have a duty of care to our neighbour or someone who could reasonably expect to be affected by our actions or omissions.

The test for establishing duty of care requires that harm

must be reasonably foreseeable, as a result of the defendant's conduct, a relationship of proximity must exist, and that it must be fair, just and reasonable to impose liability. It must also be established that there has been a breach of the duty of care. In any action, the courts will consider the standard of care that a reasonable person would have taken in the circumstances.

If the defendant failed to meet that standard, the court will then consider in the circumstances of the particular case whether the standard requires to be adjusted for any reason. Such reasons can be professional standards which a reasonable professional person may be expected to follow, in which case those standards may be applied. Common practice or guidelines can be used as appropriate standards, if it was reasonable in the circumstances to expect more than usual care because of disability or frailty on the part of the plaintiff.

In any action in negligence, it must be established that the claimant has suffered loss or damage, as a direct consequence of the defendant's breach of a duty of care.

There are two defences a defendant can plead if they are found liable.

Firstly, the claimant accepted that there was a risk of injury or loss, in which case the defendant will not be liable.

Secondly, contracts are generally drawn up describing that a particular procedure is not guaranteed to produce a required result or outcome. If a purchaser signs such a contract, they are unlikely to succeed in a claim of negligence. To summarise, the most usual definition of negligence is that it is conduct or a failure to act that breaches a duty of care. It can be broken down into three distinct elements all of which must exist to give rise to a liability to pay compensation.

1. There must be a duty owed.
2. The action or inaction needs to fall below the

standard expected of a reasonably competent person. It is this that constitutes the breach of duty.

3. The breach must cause loss, whether physical damage to a person or property, or financial loss.

Negligence can be something that occurs in everyday life, such as a local council that fails to repair a public pavement, resulting in injury to a pedestrian. Consequently, in these everyday situations, it can be difficult to sometimes know whether a duty of care was in fact owed. The test here is: "Was it foreseeable that the injured person could be injured, and is it fair, just and reasonable to impose a duty?"

Breach of Statutory Duty

Negligent acts can constitute a breach of a statutory duty. The government controls many aspects of British citizens' lives and conduct through acts of parliament and statutory regulations. If a person does not comply with any legislation or regulation that apply to the individual, then they may become liable for breach of statutory duty as well as negligence. However, breaches of statutory duty are often much easier to prove than negligence generally, because the legislation or regulations impose defined duties of care, and set out how these duties can be discharged.

A good example are the regulations that set out how workplaces should be made safe. On construction sites, if appropriate, scaffolding is not erected in accordance with the regulations to prevent falls, then any person injured by a fall is likely to be able to establish easily that there was a breach of a statutory duty by the contractors. The injured party would not have to establish what the duty was and how it was breached. The regulations in force provide all this evidence.

Contributory Negligence

If a person contributed to their own injury or loss, then the compensation payable by the person who actually caused the wrong, is liable to be reduced. For example, if a person is injured in car accident and was not wearing a seat belt, they would be held partly responsible for their own injuries. Negligence is conduct and not a state of mind, which involves an unreasonably greater risk of causing harm or damage.

Negligence has been described as: "The omission to do something which a reasonable man, guided upon those considerations which ordinarily regulate the conduct of human affairs, would do, or doing something which a prudent and reasonable man would not do".
Blyth v Birmingham Waterworks Co (1856) 11, Exch. 781.

It is not sufficient for a claimant to establish that the defendant had been careless, he must also establish that the defendant has been careless in breach of a specific legal duty to take care. However, it is a question of law whether in any particular circumstance, a duty of care exists. The law in all cases exacts a degree of care commensurate with the risk created. There are two factors in determining the magnitude of a risk; the seriousness of the injury risked, and the likelihood of the injury being in fact caused. The general principle is that before negligence can be established, it must be shown not only that the event was foreseeable but also that there is a reasonable likelihood of injury.

Proof of Negligence

The burden of proving negligence is on the claimant who alleges it. It is for the person who suffers the harm to prove that it was due to the negligence of the defendant.

Unless the claimant produces reasonable evidence that the injury or loss was caused by the defendant's negligence, there is no case to go before a jury. The claimant's evidence must go beyond pure conjecture into legal inference.

The dividing line between conjecture and inference is a difficult one. A conjecture may be plausible but it is of no legal value because it is essentially a mere guess. On the other hand, an inference in the legal sense is a reasonable deduction from the evidence and it may have the validity of legal proof.

The point of taking an action in tort, is to obtain compensation. In civil proceedings, the claimant sues the defendant. If he or she succeeds, they obtain a judgment and will be awarded a remedy to compensate the claimant for the civil wrong which the defendant has been shown, on a balance of probability, to have inflicted on the claimant.

However, there is no automatic right to compensation in tort law simply because the claimant has suffered injury. Tort law is concerned with what the defendant did not why it was done, and what the claimant suffered as a reasonably foreseeable consequence. There is no liability for negligence unless there is, in a particular case, a legal duty to take care, and this duty must be one which is owed to the claimant in person, and not merely to others.

In the absence of some existing duty, the general principle is that there is no liability for a mere omission to act. The fundamental notion appears to be that the imposition of an obligation to take positive steps for the benefit of another, requires that the other should furnish something by way of consideration. The burden of proof lies heavily on a claimant who alleges that the negligence complained of consists in an act of omission.
Kelly v Metropolitan Rly (1895) 1 QB. 944.

The law of torts does not recognise different standards of care or different degrees of negligence in different classes of cases. The sole standard is the case that would be shown is that of a reasonably careful man, and the sole form of negligence is a failure to use this amount of care. It is a negligent act to voluntarily undertake the doing of any act which can be safely done only through the possession of a special skill, unless the doer possesses or believes on reasonable grounds, that he possesses that requisite skill. It is care, not skill which is owed to the claimant. The negligence does not consist in the lack of skill, but in undertaking the work without skill.

Lewis v Carmarthenshire County Council, (1953) All ER 1025.

The Likelihood of Injury

The general principle is that before negligence can be established, it must be shown, not only that the event was foreseeable, but also that there was a reasonable likelihood of injury actually occurring. The burden of proving negligence is on the claimant who alleges it. Unless the claimant produces reasonable evidence that the accident was caused by the defendant's negligence, there is no case to go before a jury. In such cases, it is the judge's duty to enter a judgment for the defendant. In withdrawing the case from the jury, the judge does not substitute his own opinion as to the proof of negligence. He decides not that the negligence has not been proved, but that no reasonable man or jury would think it had been proved. It is to an examination of medical practice in the United Kingdom that we now turn in Chapter Two.

CHAPTER TWO:
The Development of a Health Service in the UK

Before examining the modern system of health provision in the UK, it will be helpful for readers to appreciate the historical development of the National Health Service (NHS).

The Service was established in 1948 following the passing of the first National Health Service Act in 1946. Prior to this, the public provision of health care was very limited. The Poor Law institutions were the main source of public provisions of hospital services. Additionally, these services were also provided by voluntary hospitals, usually established on a charitable basis.

The National Insurance Act of 1911 sought to provide free GP services to certain groups of workers. In 1929, the Local Government Act transferred to local authorities the responsibility for administering the poor law hospital services. However, beyond this, and until 1948, health care in the UK was a matter for private agreement between doctors and their patients.

The 1946 Act created the National Health Services (NHS), which introduced a full and comprehensive public service of health care provision. The NHS structure distinguished between the provision of primary health care services (GPs and others), hospital services (hospital boards) and community health care services (by local authorities). It was not until the National Health Service Re-Organisation Act of 1973, that community health care services were taken out of local authority control, and together with other allied medical services, were put under the control of Health Authorities. However, local authorities retained responsibility for community services involving social care provision, which included domiciliary support and residential care for the aged and infirm. It was under the Local Authority Social Services Act passed in 1970 that social and medical community services became split between local authority's health and social services departments.

It was the National Health Service Act of 1973 that created the structural pattern of Statutory Health Authorities and Area Health Authorities. The National Health Service Act of 1977 is the principal legislation setting up the NHS as it is reflected today in the UK. Under this Act, Health Authorities have a statutory duty to make arrangements for the provision of primary care services (GP services), dental services, ophthalmic services and pharmaceutical services. By 1982, the health system introduced District Health Authorities whose jurisdiction was limited to locally-defined areas of the country. The current system emerged in 1996 following the passing of the Health Authorities Act in 1995.

During the period from the 1970s through to the 1990s, there had been criticism that the NHS had become too bureaucratic in its administration and was regarded as inefficient in its delivery of services. The prime purpose in passing the Health Authorities Act in 1995 was to simplify the existing system in operation at the time. There had arisen confusion regarding the separate roles of the regional health authorities, family health service authorities, and district authorities. The 1995 Act provided an integrated authority whose main function was to provide health services for local populations.

The original National Health Service Act of 1946 placed duties on the Secretary of State for Health, to "provide a comprehensive health service". This was further enhanced by the 1977 Act. These duties were delegated to the Department of Health, who then delegated the control of health matters to the NHS Executive. This Executive is the central focus of strategic planning and policy within the NHS system. The Executive exerts significant pressure over local NHS spending by health authorities throughout the UK. One of the prime debating points of the NHS concerns the issues of cost.

NHS TRUSTS AND SERVICE PROVISION

These bodies are independent of health authorities and are formed by specific statutory instruments devolved directly from the National Health Service and Community Care Act of 1990. Whilst NHS Trusts are not under the direct control of health authorities because of the delegation of their power, they are nonetheless responsible directly to the Secretary of State for Health. These Trusts are permitted to provide NHS patients with private care provided the patient is prepared to pay the costs. They also have the power under certain circumstances to compulsory purchase land for development.

CONTROL OF MEDICAL PRACTICE

In addition to the many legal controls placed on the practice of medicine today, it is the medical profession itself that has developed internal regulation of its practising members. This can be enforced by the doctors' own union, the British Medical Association (BMA) or through the General Medical Council (GMC). Other allied professions within medicine such as nursing, have their own professional bodies controlling their practices.

THE GENERAL MEDICAL COUNCIL

The key issue as far as medical lawyers and the general public are concerned, is that the medical profession as a whole is internally accountable for their actions. For example, a doctor who is found to be lacking in performing some medical procedure will, in addition to being liable for damages to an injured party, also possibly face professional censure by the GMC. While accountability lies at the heart of public satisfaction with existing medical regulation, there is strong criticism of the nature and overall effectiveness of these disciplinary and complaint procedures.

An aggrieved patient wishing to pursue a complaint against a doctor faces a complex system of procedures to overcome. The GMC has a potentially wide power over the direction of a doctor's career. Section 36 of the Medical Act 1983, sets out the statutory powers of the GMC:

"Where a fully registered person (a) is found by the Professional Conduct Committee to have been convicted in the British Isles of a criminal offence, whether while registered or not, or (b) is judged by the Professional Conduct Committee to have been guilty of serious professional misconduct whether while so registered or not, the Committee may, if they think fit, direct that his/her name shall be erased from the register , or that his/her registration in the register be suspended during a period not exceeding 12 months, or his/her registration shall be conditional on his/her compliance during a period not exceeding three years, as specified in the requirements of the Committee".

While the GMC remains the governing body of the medical profession, its most significant public function is in ensuring that medical professionals are up to date and fit to practice. Whatever may be the overall standard of fitness, there is no doubt that the number of high profile individual instances of alleged misconduct that were exposed towards the end of the 20th century in the UK, caused both outrage and disquiet among the public. How far this was fanned by the increasingly aggressive news media, or was dictated by political expediency remains a matter for debate.

However, the fact remained that sufficient evidence accrued to provide solid grounds for review and revision of the system of control of the medical profession. A number of major incidents were disclosed and resulted in public inquiries. These included the standards of paediatric cardiac surgery at Bristol Royal Infirmary, and the retention of children's organs at Alder Hey Children's Hospital in Liverpool. Also included here were the murders of his patients by the GP Harold Shipman.

Maintaining the official register of medical practitioners is a basic function of the GMC. The purpose of the register has been to protect the public from those who have not undergone recognised medical training. However, and surprisingly, in the UK, no offence lies in an unqualified person practising medicine. The criminal offence is that of pretending to be a registered medical practitioner. A doctor's 'fitness to practice' can be questioned before a Fitness to Practice Panel on the grounds of misconduct, deficient professional performance, a conviction for or a caution following a criminal offence, on his or her physical health, and a determination that his/her fitness to practice is impaired.

A doctor whose fitness to practice is found to be impaired may be subject to erasure from the Register (except in a health case) or to suspension from practice for up to 12 months.

A doctor may appeal against a decision of the Fitness to Practice Panel, to the High Court in England and Wales, the Court of Session in Scotland, and the High Court in Northern Ireland. These appeals are allowed under Section 29 of the National Health Service Reform and Health Care Professions Act of 2002.

Supervisory regulations of the 'regulators' appears to be a feature of modern medical governance in the UK. There is the Commission for Health Improvement which is responsible for providing advice and information to, and reporting on, NHS and Primary Care Trusts. Then there is the National Institute for Clinical Excellence (NICE) which provides information on what is the best practice in medicine. Finally, there is the National Clinical Assessment Authority which provides a service to NHS bodies concerned with the performance of individual doctors. The efficacy of the General Medical Council's disciplinary powers and means of maintaining standards of competence and good practice within the profession, and protecting patients, depends on what the Council considers to be 'serious professional misconduct'.

The GMC has now recognised that 'gross negligent practice' equals misconduct. However, two constraints limit any valid interpretation of what constitutes misconduct. It must be recognised that error alone does not constitute misconduct. Even good doctors can make bad mistakes just like any other professionals, and this must be accepted as fact. The GMC can only act within the limits set by parliament and the courts.

To constitute serious professional misconduct, it must be demonstrated both that the person fell short of the standards to be expected from his or her profession, and that the failures were serious in both nature and degree. Doctors must recognise the limits of their own professional competence, and also keep their knowledge and skills up to date. However, suspicion still persists that doctors who fail patients are in all but name excused. This then raises the question are there any valid grounds for this suspicion?

It is a fact that a high degree of proof is demanded before a doctor will be found liable. The allegation levelled against a doctor must be proved beyond all reasonable doubt, the same criteria as in criminal cases. This is no different to the standard pertaining in any other professional disciplinary committee.

Patient's organisations complain about the relatively small number of cases that ever reach the Professional Conduct Committee of the GMC. This is largely due to the fact that there are in place elaborate screening procedures which seek to eliminate frivolous complaints. If a complaint relates to an NHS doctor and concerns poor practice rather than personal misconduct, the patient is referred to the NHS General Complaints procedure. Only if the doctor is found to be culpable within the NHS system, is the matter then referred to the GMC.

Within the GMC, a complaint received is examined by a Preliminary Screener. If this Screener, consulting with a lay member of the GMC considers that there is a case to answer, then the evidence is placed before the Preliminary Proceedings Committee (PPC) of the GMC. It is the PCC who then decide whether to commit the doctor for a full disciplinary hearing before the Professional Conduct Committee (PCC).

Patients do find that the proportion of complaints dismissed in the early stages of the process is suspicious. Whether there are grounds to support this suspicion is debateable. It is to an in-depth analysis of the basis for Clinical Negligence actions that we turn in Chapter Three.

CHAPTER THREE
The Basics of Clinical Negligence

The majority of claims in respect of medical injury are brought in tort, on the basis of a non-contractual wrong. The reason for this is that within the NHS, patients are not in a contractual relationship with the doctor treating them. By contrast, in the private sector, there will be a contractual relationship, so that it is possible to bring an action for damages in contract. However, in practice, there is very little difference between the two remedies, but the law of contract may provide a remedy for an express or implied warranty given by a doctor, although this would fall short of an actual guarantee.

A medical injury may have been caused to the claimant by any one or more of the medical personnel treating them. As a result, locating negligence may in some cases be a simple process. However, in others, the patient may have to choose the responsible individual or individuals from a larger group. In such a situation, these may include a GP, a hospital consultant, other hospital doctors, including the nursing staff. Locating the specific act of alleged negligence which actually caused the injury may be complicated.

The complainant may proceed directly against the doctor in question if the allegation of negligence is made against a General Practitioner (GP) who, in the UK, are solely responsible for the treatment of their patients. There can be no question of responsibility being imposed on a health authority, unless that authority has intervened in the GP's treatment of the patient. In addition, all partners in a medical practice can be held liable for the actions of one of their partners. The General Practitioner must have approved indemnity insurance cover as required by Section 9 of the Health Act 1999. This will usually be by way of membership of a medical defence society, to whom the GP can refer any claims made against them.

The Society will advise the GP and undertake any defence of its members or make a settlement of any claim. GPs are not covered by the NHS Indemnity Scheme which applies to hospital doctors. In addition, a GP is vicariously liable for the negligence of employed staff at the practice, such as nurses, receptionists and office staff. However, this does not include the acts of locum tenens or deputising doctors who are normally insured independently. However, the position changes significantly if the alleged negligence occurred after the GP referred the patient for further investigation or treatment within the NHS system. If the negligent act was committed by a health service employee, the patient has the choice of proceeding either against the identified individual, against the health authority or trust, or commence a joint action against both the trust and the individual.

However, it is usual practice to bring actions against the health authority or trust on the grounds of both expediency and convenience. The liability of the authority or trust may be based on either of two grounds, (1) the duty of a hospital to care for patients or (2) the vicarious liability of a health authority for the negligence of its employees. In the case of hospital doctors, the vast majority are direct employees of the NHS, therefore the health authority is liable for their negligence under the principle of vicarious liability. However, the employer (trust hospital) is only liable for torts committed by employees during the course of their employment.

In determining whether there has been negligence in medical treatment, the courts pursue the same lines of inquiry as they do in any other similar claim. Did the conduct of the defendant amount to a breach of the duty of care which he or she owed to the injured patient? This amounts to asking whether the standard of treatment given by the defendant fell below the standard expected of him or her by the law, and whether there was any fault in the legal sense. Fault remains the theoretical underpinning of the law in this area, until such times as strict liability can be imposed. A major difficulty for any claimant lies in the burden which falls upon him or her to prove that the defendant's negligence caused his or her injury.

STANDARD OF CARE

There have been many judicial pronouncements by the courts on the standard of care expected of a doctor. In R-v-Bateman (1925) (94 I JKB 791), the court explained that "If a person holds himself out as possessing special skill and knowledge on behalf of a patient, he owes a duty to the patient to use due caution in undertaking the treatment. The jury should not exact the highest, or very high standard, nor should they be content with a very low standard".

In other words, the doctor is not expected to be a miracle worker guaranteeing a cure, or a man of the very highest skill in his profession. This then raises another question. What standard *is* he expected to meet? J McNair, in the now familiar case in medical law Bolam-v-Friern Hospital Management Committee (1957) (2 All ER 118), said: "The test is the standard of the ordinary man exercising and professing to have that special skill. The doctor having that degree of competence expected of the ordinary skilful doctor sets the standard. He is the practitioner who follows that standard practice of his profession, or at least follows practices that would not be disapproved of by responsible opinion within the medical profession. He has a reasonably sound grasp of medical techniques, and as informed of new medical developments as the average competent doctor would expect to be".

The circumstances in which a doctor treats his or her patient will also be taken into account. A doctor working in an emergency situation and placed under great pressure, will not be expected by courts to achieve the same results as a doctor who is working in ideal conditions. This point was raised by J Mustill in the case of (Wilsher-v-Essex Area Health Authority (1987) (QB 730 at 749) where he said: "…if a person was forced by an emergency to do too many things at once, then the fact that he does one of them incorrectly, should not lightly be taken as negligent".

The reasonably skilful doctor has a duty to keep him or herself informed of major developments in medical practice. Obviously, this duty does not extend to reading everything in a particular area of medical speciality.

In the case of Cranford-v-Board of Governors of Charing Cross Hospital (1953) reported in *The Times* 8 December) the claimant had developed brachial palsy as a result of his arm being kept in a certain position during an operation. Six months prior to the operation, an article had appeared in *The Lancet*, pointing out this exact danger. However, the defendant anaesthetist against whom negligence was alleged, admitted that he had not read the article in question.

On appeal, the court eventually found in the defendant's favour. In this case, Lord Denning stated that: "It would be, I think, putting it too high a burden on a medical man to say that he has to read every article appearing in the current medical press, and it would be quite wrong to suggest that a medical man is negligent because he does not at once put into operation the suggestions which some contributor or other might make in a medical journal".

Failure to read a single article it was said may be excusable, while complete disregard of a series of warnings in the medical press, could well be evidence of negligence. In view of the rapid progress being made in many areas of medicine today, and in view of the amount of information confronting the average doctor, it is unreasonable to expect a doctor to be aware of every development in his or her particular field of expertise.

USUAL PRACTICE

The 'custom test', that is the test whereby a defendant's conduct is tested against the normal usage of his or her profession, is one that is applied in all areas of negligence law. The courts have given expression to this test in the medical context in a number of decisions.

In the important Scottish case of Hunter-v-Hanley (1955) (SC 200 at 206), there was clear endorsement of the custom test per Lord Clyde: "To establish liability by a doctor, where deviation from normal practice is alleged, three facts require to be established. First of all, it must be proved that there is an unusual and normal practice. Secondly, it must be proved that the defendant has not adopted that practice. Thirdly, it must be established that the course the doctor adopted is one which no professional man of ordinary skill would have taken if he had been acting with ordinary care".

However, this exposition of the law conceals a hurdle from the outset. It may, in many cases, be possible to prove that there is a usual and normal practice, particularly if there are published guidelines covering a particular procedure. This is a ploy which is increasingly being used in UK legislation, and which might be viewed as helpful to a claimant. On the other hand, there will obviously be disagreement as to what is the appropriate course to follow in a number of medical scenarios.

In some circumstances, the existence of two schools of thought may result in more than one option being open to a practitioner. If this is so, then what are the liability implications of choosing a course of action which a "responsible body of opinion within the profession may very well reject?" This is precisely the question that arose in the now familiar case of Bolam-v-Friern Hospital

Management Committee (1957) (2 All ER 118).

In this landmark case, the claimant had suffered fractures as a result of the administration of electro-convulsive therapy (ECT) without an anaesthetic. At the material time, there were two schools of thought on the subject of anaesthesia in such treatment. One held the view that relaxant drugs should be used, the other being that this only increased the risk.

In this particular case, the judge ruled that a doctor would not be negligent if he acted "in accordance with the practice accepted by a responsible body of medical men skilled in that particular art". Negligence would not be inferred simply because there was a body of opinion which took a contrary view. The Bolam case has been the object of sustained criticism from those who object to the implication that the medical profession itself determines what is an acceptable level of care. Critics persistently argue that doctors themselves should not determine whether conduct is negligent. This should be a matter for the courts to decide.

The House of Lords' decision in the case of Bolitho-v-Hackney Health Authority (1998) (AC 232) was regarded by some legal commentators as representing a significant departure from the decision in the Bolam case. The Bolitho case arose out of a failure on the part of a hospital doctor to examine and intubate a child experiencing respiratory distress. In this particular case, negligence derived from a failure to attend, and was not disputed. However, the problem of causation still remained to be proven. Expert evidence was led by the claimant to the effect that a reasonably competent doctor would have intubated the patient in such circumstances.

The defendant doctor had her own expert witness who stated that non-intubation was a clinically justifiable response to the situation. The defendant argued that, had she attended the child, she would not have intubated her, and that her failure to attend would not, therefore, have made any difference to the ultimate outcome.

The claim against the defendant was that the doctor's failure to attend amounted to a breach of duty of care, and resulted in "asphyxia and consequent brain damage" to the child. The defendant did admit a breach of duty. In this case, the issue for the House of Lords was whether the defendant had caused the child's injuries. It was conceded that it was negligence for a doctor not to attend the child. However, it was argued by the defendant's experts, that even if a doctor had attended, he or she would not have intubated the child and thereby avoided the child's injury being caused, therefore, it was 'but for' causation.

The House of Lords accepted the original trial judge's finding that the doctor would not have intubated the patient had she attended. However, that was not the only relevant question in this case. Causation could also be established by proving that the doctor ought to have intubated, and her failure to do this was in itself negligent. However, the case becomes more complex because expert evidence was given that supported two opposing practices; one which would have intubated the child, the other would not have done. The appeal to the House of Lords was dismissed with all the Lords in agreement.

The causation issue is important in this case in so far as it was made clear that, while the Bolam test had no relevance as to the doctor's intention, it was central to the collateral question, would she have been negligent in failing to take action?

Given that the defendant doctor had responsible support the action failed. The particular significance of this case lies in the House of Lord's support for the Court of Appeal's departure from the 'certainties of Bolam'. Rather than accepting a body of opinion simply because it was there, Lord Brown-Wilkinson held that the court must, in addition, be satisfied that the body of opinion in question rests on a logical basis.

"In particular, in cases involving, as they do so often do, the weighing of risks against benefits, the judges before accepting a body of opinion as being 'responsible' or 'respectable', will need to be satisfied that, informing their views, the experts have directed their minds to the question of comparative risks and benefits, and have reached a defensive conclusion on the matter".

Bolitho undoubtedly devalues the advantage which Bolam presented to the medical profession, but only in limited circumstances. Bolam provides some protection for the innovative or minority opinion. If this protection is removed, then the opinion which the cautious practitioner will follow will be that which involves least risk. This may well have an inhibiting effect on medical progress. Many of the advances that have been achieved in medicine have been accomplished by those who have pursued an unconventional line of therapy or inquiry.

MISDIAGNOSIS

A doctor is expected by law to use the same degree of care in making a diagnosis that is required of him or her in all dealings with his or her patients. A mistake in diagnosis will not be considered negligent if this standard of care is observed. It will be treated as one of the non-culpable and inevitable hazards of medical practice.

However, liability may be imposed when a mistake in diagnosis is made because the doctor failed to take a proper medical history of the patient, failed to conduct tests which a competent practitioner would have considered appropriate, or simply failed to diagnose a condition which would have been spotted by a competent practitioner. As a bare minimum, the doctor must examine his or her patient and pay adequate attention to the patient's medical notes, and to what the patient imparts to them. It is in this respect

that telephone diagnosis is now considered hazardous especially if the facts related by the patient are such as raise the doctor's suspicion that can only be allayed by a clinical examination.
(Barrett-v-Chelsea and Kensington Hospital Management Committee (1969), 1 QB 428).

One of the problems in determining whether there has been a mistake in diagnosis, turns on deciding what investigative techniques need to be used in a particular case. Routine laboratory tests must be considered if symptoms suggest their use is required. In those cases where a doctor is doubtful about a diagnosis, good practice may require that the patient be referred to a specialist for further consideration.

NEGLIGENCE IN TREATMENT

The most important distinction to be made is that between a medical mistake which the law regards as excusable and a mistake which would amount to negligence. In the former case, the court will accept that ordinary human fallibility precludes liability, while in the latter, the conduct of the defendant is considered to have strayed beyond the bounds of what is expected of the 'reasonably skilled or competent doctor'. This issue came before the courts most classically in the case of Whitehouse-v-Jordan (1981) (1 All ER 267).

In this case, negligence was alleged on the part of the obstetrician who, it was claimed, had pulled too hard in a trial of forceps delivery, and had thereby caused the child's head to become wedged, with consequent asphyxia and brain damage. The trial judge held that, although the decision to perform a trial of forceps was a reasonable one, the defendant had in fact pulled too hard and was therefore negligent.

Many historic cases deal with items of operating equipment left inside patients following surgery. In these, generally termed 'swab cases', the allocation of liability is made according to the principles laid down in the law on this point, in the decision in the case of Mahon-v-Osborne (1939) (2 KB4).

In this case, as in subsequent decisions, the courts have shown themselves unlikely to dictate to doctors in a hard and fast way, the exact procedures that should have been used towards the end of an operation, in order to ensure that no foreign bodies are left inside the patient. At some time, however, it is clear that the law requires that there should be some sort of set procedures adopted in order to minimise the possibility of this occurrence.

Overall responsibility to see that swabs and other items are not left in the patient rests entirely on the surgeon. He or she is not entitled to delegate the matter entirely to a nurse. This point was particularly emphasised in the Mahon case.

THE PROBLEM OF TRAINEE MEDICAL STAFF

The degree of expertise possessed by a medical practitioner obviously depends to a considerable extent on his or her experience. The argument has been put forward that the standard of competence of a newly qualified doctor will be less than that expected of an experienced practitioner. However, this is not the expectation of the law; and the strict application of the Bolam test would lead the courts to expect the doctor to show that degree of skill which would be shown by the reasonably competent professional.

This is an objective standard, therefore it is irrelevant whether the doctor is recently qualified or not, as regards an alleged incident of negligence. It should, therefore, make no difference to the way in which the doctor's conduct is assessed.

This particular problem was considered in the case of Wilsher-Essex Area Health Authority (1987) (QB 730 3 All ER 801). The claimant (child) had been born prematurely and had been admitted to a specialised neonatal intensive care unit. Extra oxygen was administered by a junior hospital doctor who made an error in monitoring arterial oxygen tension. It was claimed that this could have caused the virtually blinding condition of retrolental fibroplasia, which did occur. It was argued by the defendants, that the standard of care expected of the junior doctor was not the same as that of his or her experienced counterpart.

Extensive use, it was said, by the hospital had to be made of recently qualified medical and nursing staff, and it was unavoidable that such staff should have to learn on the job. It was further argued that it would be impossible for public medicine to operate properly without such arrangements and to do otherwise, would not be in the interests of patients.

In the Court of Appeal, the majority of the judges maintained that the public were entitled to expect a reasonable standard of competence in their medical attendants. However, the decision of Lord Justice Mostill made it clear that he, at least, was prepared to define the standard of care according to the requirements of the particular post.

An inexperienced doctor occupying a post in a unit which offered specialised service would, accordingly, need that degree of expertise expected of a reasonably competent person occupying that post. The defendant's actual hospital rank; house officer, registrar or consultant, would not be relevant in the determination. Hospital authorities cannot rely too much on junior employees because the principle of vicarious liability prevents this.

For example, a consultant could be held to be negligent

were he or she delegates responsibilities to a junior doctor in the knowledge that the junior was incapable of performing his or her duties properly, due to the lack of experience. However, a junior to whom responsibility has been delegated, must carry out his or her duties as instructed by his or her superior to avoid liability. If he or she chooses to deviate from specific instructions, then he or she will be placed in a risky position in the event that anything goes wrong. However, there may be circumstances in which he or she is entitled to depart from instructions; obedience to manifestly wrong instructions might itself be construed as negligent in some cases.

THE PRINCIPLE OF 'RES IPSA LOQUITOR'

Because it may be difficult in many personal injury actions to establish negligence on the part of the defendant, Claimants occasionally have recourse to the principle of 'res ipsa loquitor', which translated from the Latin reads 'the facts speak for themselves'. This principle does not shift the onus of proof to the defendant, but what it does do, is to give rise to an inference of negligence, on the defendant's part. If the defendant cannot then rebut this inference of negligence, the claimant will then have established his or her case. It naturally follows from this that it will be considerably easier for the claimant to succeed in his or her action when the principle is applied.

The classic case here is probably that of Cassidy-v-Ministry of Health (1951) (2 KB 343). The claimant went into hospital for an operation to remedy Dupuytren's Contracture of two fingers, and came out with four stiff fingers. Lord Justice Denning at the Appeal hearing, expressed the view that the claimant was quite entitled to say: "I went into hospital to be cured of two stiff fingers, I have come out with four stiff fingers and my hand is useless. That should not have happened. Explain it if you can".

The principle can apply only where the claimant is unable to identify the precise nature of the negligence, and where no explanation of the way in which the injury came to be inflicted has been offered by the defendant.

The injury itself must be of such a kind as does not normally happen in the circumstances, unless there is negligence. The principle's application in medical cases may still be applicable because of the difficulty the ordinary claimant sometimes experiences establishing the cause of an injury sustained during technical procedures of which he or she possesses little understanding. It may also be seen as a potential corrective to the tendency of the medical profession as a whole, to close ranks when one of their number is accused of negligence. However, the courts remain generally reluctant to apply the principle.

An unsuccessful attempt to raise the principle was made in the case of Ludlow-v-Swindon Health Authority (1989) (1 Med LR 104). In this case it was stressed that the claimant had to establish facts which, if unexplained, would give rise to an inference of negligence. The claimant claimed to have regained consciousness during a caesarean section operation, and to have experienced intense pain. She failed however, to establish that the pain arose at a stage during which halothane should have been administered. There was, accordingly, the inference of negligence in the administration of anaesthetic.

However, there are cases where the injuries sustained by the patient are of such a nature that there is inescapable inference of negligence. In Glass-v-Cambridge Heath Authority (1995) (6 Med LR 91) the patient suffered brain damage as a result of suffering a heart attack under a general anaesthetic. The court held that this was not an event which normally would be expected to happen in the circumstances, and that the onus therefore transferred to the defendant to provide an explanation of the event which was consistent with the absence of negligence.

CAUSATION: THE RELATIONSHIP OF CAUSE AND EFFECT

The majority of cases of medical negligence involve something going wrong as a result of a medical mistake. The claimant's problem is to prove that what was done, or not done, amounts to actionable negligence. However, proving negligence by a doctor, does not conclude the case in the claimant's favour. He or she must also show that their injury, or condition, was caused by the doctor's negligence. They must prove what in law is termed 'causation'.

In practice, proving causation is often the most problematic aspect of a patient's claim. The difficulties of causation in medical malpractice cases fall into two main groups.

First, can the patient convince the court that it was the relevant negligence that caused their injury, rather than the progress of an original disease or condition?

Second, how should the courts proceed when the essence of a claim is, not that clinical negligence caused any additional injury to the patient, but that negligence deprived him or her of a chance of full recovery from their original disease or condition?

The burden of proving causation, rests on the claimant alone, and does not move to the defendant even though negligence has been proved or even admitted. What is crucial for the claimant in any action, is the quality of the expert scientific evidence, presented on their behalf. That evidence must at the very least demonstrate that it is more likely than not, that the defendant's negligence materially contributed to the claimant's condition, or materially increased the risk that the claimant would succumb to such a condition.

Where the scientific evidence is ambivalent or suggests

a competing or different cause, for the claimant's condition, any action for negligence would fail. Uncertainty about causation is likely to be common in many claims that essentially relate to whether the defendant's negligence caused or exacerbated disease. When a claimant complains not of some new injury inflicted by the defendant, but of a lost chance of recovery, their claim is even more difficult to prove.

In the case of Hotson-v-East Berkshire Health Authority (1987) (2 All ER 909-HL) the claimant, a schoolboy of 13, fell heavily from a rope on which he had been swinging, to the ground 4 metres below. He was taken to hospital, where his knee was x-rayed, but no injury was revealed. No further examination was made and he was sent home. Five days later, the boy was taken back to the same hospital and an injury to his hip joint was diagnosed and swiftly and correctly treated. The boy suffered a condition known as avascular necrosis. This condition, caused by a restriction of the blood supply in the region of the original injury, leads to misshaping of the joint, disability and pain, and later in life almost certainly brings on osteoarthritis in the joint.

The claimant's disability might have ensued from the accident in any case, but there was a 25% chance that given the correct treatment immediately, the claimant might have avoided disability and made a nearly full recovery.

The defendant hospital admitted negligence in failing to diagnose and treat the complainant's injury on his first visit. Both parties agreed that prompt treatment would have offered a 25% chance of avoiding permanent disability. The trial judge awarded the boy 25% of full compensation for his condition. That is a sum of money to compensate him for a 25% lost chance of making a full recovery. The House of Lords questioned this judgment. Their Lordships held that the claimant had failed to prove that it was more likely than not that the avascular necrosis resulting from the negligent delay in treatment, because there was a 75% chance he would have suffered from avascular necrosis in any event even if this treatment had been given promptly. To recover damages for the avascular necrosis, the claimant required to establish a better than 50/50 likelihood that 'but for' the negligent delay in treatment, he would have made an uncomplicated recovery from his original injury.

Had he succeeded in doing so, he would have been entitled to 100% compensation for his disability.

Expert evidence suggests that the relevant negligent mismanagement of, or delay in, treatment diminished his prospects of recovery by an ascertainable percentage. For example, if a doctor negligently failed to diagnose cancer, and a further period elapsed before a proper diagnosis was made and treatment begun, might the patient be allowed to recover damages for diminished prospects of survival or recovery? Perhaps at the time when the diagnosis should have been made, the patient would have had a 75% chance of recovery. However, by the time it was in fact made, that chance had diminished to 50%.

Such a case differs from Hotson in this way. On the evidence available in Hotson, no one could say whether or not 'but for' the relevant negligence the complainant would or would not have suffered avascular necrosis at all. In the example given of the unfortunate cancer patient, scientific and statistical evidence strongly indicates that 'but for' the relevant negligence, the patient would have enjoyed a much greater chance of prolonged survival.

PRIVATE PATIENTS

A patient who pays for treatment enters into a contract with his or her doctor, and they are free to set the terms of that contract. However, the doctor cannot exempt him or herself from liability for any in injury caused to his or her patient arising from his or her negligence. There is rarely a written contract between them. The terms of this contract will be implied from their relationship. This usually means that the doctor undertakes a duty of care toward the patient. His or her duty of care to the patient is no different from that duty to a patient in the NHS.

This raises the question could a doctor in private practice be found to have contracted to guaranteed the desired outcome of a specific treatment?

This situation could never happen in the NHS. The doctor can only be liable in tort for a failure of care. However, only rarely would a private doctor be found to have guaranteed a result in contract. Where a patient is ill and seeks a cure, unless the doctor foolishly and expressly promises success in his or her treatment; no court will infer any terms other than the particular doctor will exercise skill and care.

CRIMINAL LIABILITY

Negligence is normally a matter for the civil and not the criminal law. However, the situation changes if the victim dies. Gross negligence which causes death can lead to a criminal conviction for manslaughter. In such a case, much more than ordinary negligence needs to be proved. Criminal liability requires more than the degree of negligence required to establish civil liability. The doctor must be shown to have demonstrated such disregard for the life and safety of others as to amount to a crime against the state, and conduct deserving of punishment.

The conduct involved in the relevant cases have ranged from, at one extreme, complete indifference and total recklessness, to mere incompetence at the other. In the case of R-v-Adomako (1991) (5 Med LR 277) an anaesthetist failed to notice the fact that his patient was in distress when this would have been glaringly obvious to any competent practitioner. There was conflicting evidence on the question of whether the accused was out of the theatre at the time, if he had been, and if there had been a failure on his part to make adequate arrangements for the monitoring of the patient, then that would have amounted to a degree of recklessness which was deserving of punishment. If, however, he was merely incompetent, it could be more difficult to argue for his conviction of manslaughter. Undoubtedly, in such cases, professional sanctions would be required.

This case was heard on appeal in 1993 when it was held that the proper test in manslaughter cases based on breach of duty was that of gross negligence rather than recklessness. Dr Adomako's appeal failed but he carried his case to the House of Lords where his conviction was upheld.

GENERAL PRACTICE

Legal problems concerning patients and their general practitioners appear less prevalent than claims against hospital doctors. However, malpractice actions against GPs are becoming more common but still lower than those against hospital trusts. There appear to be several reasons for this obvious imbalance. NHS arrangement for general practice and the constant quality of care offered by the great majority of GPs are such that despite obvious exceptions which are still relatively rare, they enjoy high esteem among their patients. Patients have traditionally enjoyed a longstanding personal relationship with their local GP. A mistake is more likely to be forgiven and forgotten in the context of a GPs continuing care than in an impersonal hospital setting.

DUTY TO ATTEND

A frequent complaint about GPs is that patients have difficulty getting appointments or home visits, and that, in some practices, receptionists take it upon themselves to decide when and if, someone can see a doctor. What exactly is the GPs duty to attend his or her patients, and who in law are his or her patients?

GPs terms of service provide that a doctors' patients are those who are accepted on the individual doctor's practice list. Provision is made to ensure that no patient is ever without a GP. The doctors' patients also include persons accepted as temporary residents and persons to whom he or she may be requested to give treatment which is immediately required owing to an accident or other emergency at any place within his or her practice area.

Wherever an NHS patient goes, he or she should be able to see a GP. For example, if a patient falls ill on holiday and can get to a doctor, they can go temporarily onto the local doctor's list. Is there any obligation directly to the patient? Could a patient sue if their condition deteriorated because they were denied treatment?

The GP has a continuing duty to the patients on his or her list. In a dire emergency, a patient can call on and count on any GP practice in the area to come to their aid. A failure to attend such a patient where a competent GP would recognise the need for attendance is as much a breach of duty as giving wrong and careless treatment.

Patients accepted as temporary residents by a GP are in the same position for as long as they are registered with a GP. Emergency patients within a GP practice area, when a GP is on duty, are classed as a 'foreseeable class of persons' within the NHS, whereby the GP has undertaken a duty, and that duty should be not merely a moral one, but also a legal one.

A patient suing a GP will find that their problems

commence when they seek to prove as they must, that the GPs failure to treat them was negligent.

Some patients make intolerable demands on their doctor. The doctor is not obliged to respond immediately to every call. He or she has to exercise their judgment regarding priority. A GP's terms of service will require that they provide treatment during approved hours, or if they operate an appointment scheme, that the patient is offered an appointment within a reasonable time. If the patient's condition so requires, the doctor must visit the patient at home.

GPs are responsible for their staff and must ensure that their service as well as the doctor's own is efficient. The doctors' liability for their staff is absolute.

PROTOCOLS AND GUIDELINES

It appears that the in-words in medical practice today are evidence-based medicine and clinical governance. Within the NHS, the government seeks to ensure that treatment provided to patients is soundly based on good practice derived from concrete evidence.

The Health Act 1999 imposes on Primary Care Trusts and Hospital Trusts, a duty to monitor and improve quality of health care provided (sections 18-25 of the act). The National Institute for Clinical Excellence (NICE) is expressly instructed to investigate medical practice and provide guidelines of good practice. As a result, evidence of good practice as defined by protocol and guidelines, will clearly play a significant role in any claim of clinical negligence. Does this mean that any doctor deviating from official guidelines will be proven negligent? Some doctors fear that guidelines enforced by courts will lead to a tick-box approach to patient care.

Doctors would obviously cease to exercise professional judgment based on the needs and circumstances of the individual patient. Quite clearly, this should never be allowed to happen. Where departure from the guidelines can be justified in the interests of the patient, the doctor clearly discharges his or her duty of care. Guidelines will offer some evidence of what constitutes proper treatment for a patient's condition. However, evidence that a patient requires a different mode of care, is not excluded by the presence of such general guidelines.

CHAPTER FOUR:
Consent to Medical Treatment

THE THEORY OF AUTONOMY

The word 'autonomy' is derived from the Greek 'auitos' meaning 'self' and 'nomos' meaning 'rule'. Personal autonomy can be defined as 'self-rule' free from both controlling interference by others, and from limitations such as inadequate understanding which prevents meaningful choice. An autonomous individual acts freely and in accordance with a self-chosen plan.

By contrast, a person of diminished autonomy is in some respect controlled by others, or incapable of deliberating or acting on the basis of his or her own desires and plans. Virtually, all theories of autonomy agree that two conditions are essential for true autonomy. These are liberty (independence from controlling influences) and agency (the capacity for intentional personal action).

Within the context of medical practice, there is a fundamental obligation to ensure that patients have the right to choose, as well as the right to accept or decline information. Consequently, forced information or evasive disclosure are inconsistent with this obligation.

Health professionals should, as a matter of routine, always inquire in general terms about their patients' wishes to receive information and make decisions. The fundamental requirement here is to respect an individual patient's autonomous choices. Respect for autonomy is not an 'optional extra', it is a professional obligation.

Autonomous choice is a right, not a duty imposed on patients. The basic paradigm of autonomy in medical practice is express consent. Consent to a medical procedure is often implicit or implied. However, consent should refer to an individual's actual choices, and not to presumptions about choices the individual patient would or should make.

However, a significant number of patients are not competent to give valid consent. Inquiries regarding competence mainly focus on whether patients are capable psychologically or legally, of adequate decision-making. The concept of competence in decision-making has close ties to that of autonomy itself. Patients are competent to make a decision if they have the capacity to understand the material information being given and to make a considered judgment about the information in the light of their own values, to intend a certain outcome, and to communicate freely their wishes to health care professionals.

In the medical context, a person is usually considered competent if able to understand a specific procedure, to deliberate regarding its major risks and benefits, and to reach a decision based on this deliberation. If a patient lacks any of these capacities, then his or her competence to decide consent or refuse, is thrown into doubt.

Virtually, all prominent medical codes of practice hold that doctors must obtain the informed consent of patients to any significant intervention. However, some observers attempt to reduce the idea of 'informed consent' to 'shared decision-making' between doctor and patient, so that, 'informed consent' and 'mutual decision-making' are regarded as synonymous. However, legally, 'informed consent' cannot be reduced to 'shared decision-making'.

This is because an 'informed consent' is essentially an individual person's autonomous authorisation for a medical intervention. A patient must do more that express agreement or comply with a proposal. He or she must authorise something through an act of informed voluntary consent.

'Informed consent' should comprise competence, disclosure, understanding, voluntariness and consent. Therefore, a patient gives an 'informed consent' to an intervention if he or she is competent to act, through sufficient disclosure which he or she fully comprehends; acts voluntarily and finally consents to the intervention.

The obligation on the part of doctors to disclose information to patients is regarded as a necessary condition of informed consent. Civil litigation has emerged over informed consent because of injury sustained that was negligently caused by a doctor's failure to disclose. Without an adequate way for doctors to deliver information, many patients will have an inadequate basis for decision-making, which is a prerequisite of consent.

Doctors are generally obliged to describe a core set of information which should comprise those salient facts that patients consider to be material in deciding whether to refuse or consent to a proposed intervention. However, there have emerged two competing standards of disclosure of information; the 'professional practice standard' and the 'reasonable person' standard.

The professional practice standard holds that customary medical practices determine adequate disclosure. That is, professional custom within a medical practice. This establishes the amount and kind of information to be disclosed to patients. In effect, disclosure, like treatment, is a task which belongs solely to doctors because of their professional expertise and commitment to their patients' welfare.

However, there are difficulties in that the professional practice standard of disclosure subverts the right of autonomous choice by the patients themselves. Decisions for or against medical care are essentially the province of the patient and not the doctor.

Under the reasonable person standard, it must be determined that the information to be disclosed to a patient is by reference to a hypothetical reasonable person. However, under this standard, the determination of informational needs shifts from the doctor back to the patient. In this way, doctors may be found guilty of negligent disclosures.

Under this standard, it is difficult for doctors to implement the standard because they have to project what a reasonable patient would wish to know, Patients usually should understand at least what a doctor believes they require in order to authorise an intervention. To this end, diagnoses, prognoses, the nature and purpose of the intervention, alternatives, risks and benefits are all essential constituents of adequate disclosure. Unless agreement exists about these essential features of what is authorised, there can be no assurance that a patient has, in fact, made an autonomous decision.

Some studies have uncovered difficulties in patients' processing information about risks. Some ways of framing information can be so misleading that both health professionals and patients alike, misconstrue the context. For example, choices between risky alternatives can be heavily influenced by whether the same risk information is presented as providing a gain or an opportunity for a patient, or as constituting a loss or a reduction of opportunity.

These framing effects reduce understanding with direct implications for autonomous choice. If a misperception prevents a person from adequately understanding the risk of death, and this risk is material to a patient's decision-making, then the patient's choice of surgery does not reflect a substantial understanding, and, therefore, does not qualify as an autonomous authorisation of consent.

The common law recognised the principle of autonomy, that every person has the right to have their bodily integrity protected against invasion by others. The seriousness with which the law views any invasion of physical integrity is based on the strong moral conviction that everyone has the right of self-determination with regard to their body.

Unless there is consent to an act of touching by another,

such an act will constitute battery for which damages may be awarded. It is the affront to bodily integrity which makes the conduct actionable. No actual physical harm need arise. Therefore, every touching of a patient by way of medical treatment is potentially a battery.

It is the patient's consent, either informed or implied, which makes the touching legally innocuous. Is consent always needed? As a general rule, medical treatment should not proceed unless the doctor has first obtained the patient's consent. This consent may be implied, as it is when the patient presents him or herself to the doctor for examination and acquiesces in the suggested routine.

This principle applies in the majority of cases but there are limited circumstances in which a doctor may be entitled to proceed without consent. Non-voluntary treatment is that which is given when the patient is not in a position to have or express any views as to his or her management. Treatment in the absence of consent is more easily justified in such circumstances.

These include first, when the patient is incapable of giving consent by reason of unconsciousness. Second, when the patient is a minor, and finally when the patient's state of mind is such as to render a consent or refusal invalid.

When an unconscious patient is admitted to hospital, the casualty officer may argue that his or her consent could be implied or presumed on the grounds that if he or she were conscious, they would probably consent to their life being saved in this way. An alternative route would be to apply the 'necessity' principle.

It is widely recognised in both criminal and civil law that there are occasions when acting out of necessity legitimates an otherwise wrongful act. The basis of the principle is that acting unlawfully is justified if the good effect outweighs the consequences of adhering strictly to the letter of the law. Therefore, the doctor is justified and should not have criminal or civil liability imposed upon him or her, if the value which the doctor seeks is of greater weight than the wrongful act he or she performs. Necessity is a viable defence to any proceedings for non-consensual treatment where an unconscious patient is involved and there is no known objection to treatment.

However, such treatment must not be more extensive than what is required by the demands of the situation. A doctor cannot take advantage of an unconscious patient to perform procedures which are not essential for the patient's immediate survival.

In the case of Williamson v East London and City Health Authority (1997) (41 BMLR 85) the plaintiff consented to removal and replacement of a leaking breast implant. The condition at operation was found to be more serious that had been anticipated. A subcutaneous mastectomy was performed.

The judge, Butterfield J, ruled that consent to the more serious procedure had not been given and that the plaintiff would not have agreed to it had she been given the opportunity. Damages of £20,000 were awarded despite the fact that the court agreed that the operation would have been required at some time in the future. Guidance on obtaining consent in the UK was provided to all health care professionals by the Department of Health in 2001. Uniform consent forms have now been in use in the NHS since 1990.

PROXY CONSENT AND THE CONSENT OF MINORS

Proxy consents are valid only when the patient has given express authority to another person to give or withhold consent on a patient's behalf or when the law invests a person with such authority. The commonest example would be that of a patient and child. When proxy consent of this sort is available, the person vested with the power must exercise it reasonably.

A common occasion on which parents refuse to give consent to the medical treatment of their children is when they disapprove of it for religious reasons. A doctor attempting to administer life-saving treatment such as a blood transfusion to the child against the wishes of the parents, could rely upon the necessity principle. The current medical climate is such that a decision taken in good faith and in the best interests of a child would, except in unusual circumstances, be upheld by the courts.

In such a situation, it is also possible for the medical advisers to initiate care proceedings or to apply for a specific order. An alternative approach would be to invite the High Court to exercise its inherent jurisdiction, and to negate the parental decision because that power had been exercised unreasonably. In the case of R-v-O, (a minor) (1993) (2 FLR 149) it was held that the inherent jurisdiction of the High Court, by way of the Children Act 1989 section 100, was the most appropriate framework within which to consider a contested issue relating to emergency treatment for a child.

THE DANGERS OF PROCEEDING WITHOUT CONSENT

Non-consensual medical treatment entitles a patient to sue for damages for the battery which is committed. It is also possible to base a claim on the tort of negligence, the theory being that the doctor has been negligent in failing to obtain the consent of the patient. An action of battery arises when the plaintiff has been touched in some way by the defendant, and when there has been no consent, express or implied to such touching. All the plaintiff needs to establish in such an action, is that the defendant wrongfully touched him or her.

However, the problem in negligence actions based on a lack of consent, is that of causation. The court must be satisfied that the defendant's failure to obtain the valid consent of the patient was, in fact, the cause of the patient's injury. To satisfy this requirement, the patient must prove that he or she would not have given their consent had they had the information of which they were allegedly deprived.

There are several ways by which the strength of a plaintiff's case can be assessed. The first involves purely subjective judgment, what would that particular patient have considered to be adequate information?

An alternative objective approach is to postulate a standard based on a reasonable patient. Would the reasonable patient have given their consent when confronted with full information of the risks and difficulties of the procedure in question? If the answer is "Yes", then it may be inferred that the plaintiff would have consented.

Informed consent introduced a new element into medical treatment. It is now no longer a simple matter of consent to a technical assault; consent must now be based on a knowledge of the nature, risks, consequences and alternatives associated with the proposed procedure or treatment.

What needs to be disclosed? A person should not be exposed to a risk of damage unless he or she has agreed to that risk. They cannot properly agree to, or make a choice between risks, in the absence of factual information. The two problems to be resolved are, by what general standard should the information be judged, and to what extent must or should particular details be divulged?

The general standards available are described as the 'patient standard' and the 'professional standard'. In the former standard, given a rational patient, the doctor must reveal all the relevant facts as to what he or she intends to do. It is not for the doctor to determine what the patient should or should not hear. Obviously, there must be some medical assessment of what is, or is not significant, but apart from the exclusion of irrelevant materials, the patient should be as fully informed as possible, so that they can make up their mind in the light of all the relevant circumstances.

However, this approach can be criticised on the grounds that it leaves little scope for the exercise of clinical judgment by the doctor. It is for this reason that even those dedicated to patient autonomy, will allow the doctor the therapeutic privilege to withhold information which would merely serve to distress or confuse the patient. It follows that, whichever standard is adopted, litigation based on inadequate information may be taken in negligence.

Given a patient standard, the quality of information will be judged from the viewpoint of the prudent or the particular patient. Under the professional standard, it will be that of the prudent doctor.

The choice between a patient standard and a professional standard is a difficult one. There must be respect for the patient's legitimate interest in knowing to what he or she is subjecting themselves to, but at the same time, there will clearly be cases where a paternalistic approach is appropriate.

A final point about the nature of the principle of informed consent relates to patient understanding. The focus of the concept is on information given supposedly to further the autonomy of the patient. But the consequent implication is that the health care professional has fulfilled their duty once they have proffered the information. A much narrower interpretation, however, ignores consideration of the patient's ability to assimilate and analyse the information.

If it is not also part of the doctor's duty to ensure at least a degree of understanding on the part of the patient, he can discharge his duty by offering information in a way that results in the enhancement of the patient's autonomy. It is a fallacy to make consent forms longer and more detailed in an attempt to meet the requirements of the law for at least two reasons. First, this is likely to hinder rather than promote patient understanding, and second, because a signed consent form has, in any case, no binding validity.

It merely serves as some evidence that consent has been obtained, but this can always be rebutted if contrary evidence demonstrates that the patient was uncomprehending, and did not truly provide his or her voluntary consent.

Two specific aspects of the information issue are confirmed as a result of the Sidaway Case. The first is that material risks of a procedure must be disclosed, subject only to therapeutic privilege, which a doctor might be required to justify. Second, the fact that the patient asks questions revealing concerns about the risk would make the doctor aware that the patient did, in fact, attach significance to the risk.

It is also clear from Sidaway there must be a particularly good reason which the doctor would have to justify for failing to answer such questions as the patient puts, and there may be a strict obligation to do so. In the case, Lord Bridge held that

"When questioned specifically by a patient of apparently sound mind about risks involved in a particular treatment proposed, a doctor's duty must, in my opinion, be to answer both truthfully and as fully as the questioner requires".

(Sidaway v Board of Governors of the Bethlehem Royal Hospital and the Maudsley Hospital, (1984) (QB 493).

THE SIDAWAY CASE

For consent to be valid, the patient must be told what operation or procedure is to be performed and why it is to be done. The doctor certifies on the consent form that he or she has explained the proposed procedure to the patient. This raises the question, what exactly must the doctor explain?

All surgery under general anaesthetic carries a risk. Patients have argued that if they are not informed of the risks inherent in an operation, then they have inadequate information on which to make a proper decision and, therefore, cannot be said to have granted real consent to the procedure. If informed consent was not given in a particular case, a claim in battery should be. Alternatively, they argue that if a claim in battery does not lie, they ought to be able to sue for negligence.

A doctor's duty of care encompasses giving adequate information and advice. If the patient has been given inadequate information, and the patient agreed to a risky procedure from which injury ensued, the doctor is responsible for that damage.

For several years, following an accident at work, Mrs Sidaway had endured persistent pain in her right arm and shoulder. Later the pain spread to her left arm also. In 1960, she became the patient of Mr Falconer, an eminent neurosurgeon at the Maudsley Hospital. An operation relieved the pain for a while but by 1973 Mrs Sidaway was once more in pain. In October 1974, she was admitted to the Maudsley Hospital and Mr Falconer diagnosed pressure on a nerve root as the cause of her pain. He decided to operate to relieve the pressure and Mrs Sidaway gave her consent to surgery.

As a result of that operation, Mrs Sidaway became severely disabled by partial paralysis. Mrs Sidaway sued both Mr Falconer and the Maudsley Hospital. She did not suggest that the operation had been performed otherwise than skilfully and carefully. Her complaint was that the operation to which she agreed involved two specific risks over and above the risk inherent in any surgery under general anaesthesia. These were damage to a nerve root, assessed about a 2% risk, and damage to the spinal cord, assessed at less than 1% risk. Unfortunately for Mrs Sidaway, the second risk materialised and she suffered partial paralysis. She maintained that Mr Falconer never warned her of the risk of injury to the spinal cord.

Throughout the long and expensive litigation, Mrs Sidaway's greatest handicap was that Mr Falconer died before the action came to court. Consequently, the courts were deprived of vital evidence as to what exactly the patient was told by her surgeon and what reasons, if any, he had for withholding information from her.

The case had to proceed from the inference drawn by the trial judge in the High Court, that Mr Falconer would have followed his customary practice which was, he would have warned Mrs Sidaway in general terms of the possibility of injury to a nerve root, but would have said nothing about any risk of damage to the spinal cord.

Ten years after the operation that left Mrs Sidaway paralysed, and seven years after Mr Falconer's death, the case reached the House of Lords. The judge dismissed the plaintiff's claim at the original trial and the Court of Appeal affirmed the judge's decision. On further appeal to the House of Lords, the majority view was given by Lords Bridge, Templeman and Keith, and the appeal was dismissed, the overall decision was that the defendant (Mr Falconer) was not liable.

It was emphasised that the practice of not discussing a particular risk inherent in an operation prior to treatment was a clinical matter. Lord Bridge also considered that there would be "circumstances when the provision of information would be so obviously necessary to an informed choice, that no prudent medical man would fail to make it".

This would be so, even if non-disclosure was common professional practice in a particular area of medicine. A piece of information is obviously necessary if its provision will be material to the decision-making process. According to Lord Scarman in Sidaway there were four key principles of the doctrine of informed consent.

(1) It was a basic concept that an individual of adult years and sound mind, has a right to choose what shall happen to his or her body.

(2) The consent is the informed exercise of a choice and that entails an opportunity to evaluate knowledgeably, the options available, and the risks attendant on each.

(3) The doctor must, therefore, disclose all material risks; what risks are material is determined by the 'prudent patient' test. This test uses as its template, what the reasonable patient, in the plaintiff's position, would attach significance to in coming to a decision on treatment advice given.

(4) There is, however, a therapeutic privilege for the doctor to withhold information, which it is considered would prove a psychological detriment to the patient.

A successful allegation that the level of pre-operative disclosure fell below the legal standard expected, will mean nothing if the patient cannot show on the balance of probabilities that he or she would not have undertaken treatment if informed of the risk that has become a reality.

There are a number of ways that the law could deal with this factual issue. The court could adopt a subjective test of causation, and simply ask: Would this plaintiff have gone through with the operation knowing the risk? However, the problem with adopting such a simple test is that in reality, every plaintiff injured by a risk inherent in the operation that was performed would say: "If I had known of the risk, I would have refused the operation".

This would be a typical reaction to the distress of injury and the fact that they may be one of the small number that did in fact, go wrong.

At the other end of the spectrum, one could adopt a

reasonable patient test and ask: "Would a reasonably prudent patient have consented to go through an operation having been informed of the risk?"

In any trial, the judge can use personal experience, as an actual or potential patient to consider whether the patient would have gone through with the operation. However, the disadvantages lie in the fact that while the reasonable patient might well have still gone through with the operation, the particular plaintiff, because of some personal reason, would not have done so if told.

The essence of the reasonable patient analysis of causation is that it is objective whereas the traditional test for causation in negligence is subjective. The power of the medical profession to decide on the level of disclosure of information to patients appears both undesirable as a matter of English medical law at present, and increasingly anomalous. The standard of information disclosure necessary for informed consent on the part of the patient, is once more decided by the medical profession, acquiesced in by the judiciary, and therefore, out of the patient's hands.

In 1954, Denning, LJ, invoked the principle that the 'therapeutic lie', the lie that is supposed to protect a patient from worry, was legally permissible. That view still predominates in Britain today. Consequently, medical law relating to the disclosure of information is not 'good law'.

A good medical law is one which has the objective of autonomy, and it is also one that promotes truth telling. The decision of the medical law courts in Britain do neither.

CHAPTER FIVE:
Clinical Negligence Litigation

This chapter introduces the reader to the process of civil litigation. First and foremost, practical problems confront the patient. How can he or she fund a lawsuit? Whom should they sue? How quickly must they act? How do you prove negligence? What levels of compensation is available?

There are some observers in the UK who contend that the country faces a malpractice crisis and advance evidence for this contention. They maintain that the number of claims being made have escalated; that doctors are being held negligent on unfair grounds, the cost of compensation awards to patients is becoming prohibitive to the NHS, and as a result, doctors are now practising defensive medicine.

This is when a doctor will choose treatment for the patient which is considered to be legally safe, to ensure he or she will not be sued by the patient, even though the treatment may not necessarily be the best option for the patient.

This contention of increasing clinical negligence cases is destroying the doctor/patient relationship. The inevitable fall-out of these negative factors is that young aspiring doctors are being driven away from those medical specialities which are considered to be high risk areas for negligence claims.

Assessing the evidence for and against the existence of a malpractice crisis in the UK is a difficult undertaking. For the year 2021-2022, the total NHS budget in the UK was £190 billion. Negligence claims accounted for approximately 7% of the total annual budget.

The total negligence claims received by NHS Resolution in 2021 was 13,351. The most claim areas of medicine in 2021-2022 were:

Emergency Medicine	1,233
Orthopaedics	1,203
Obstetrics	1,055
General Surgery	755
Gynaecology	751

Source: resolution.nhs.uk.

The cost of clinical negligence claims is a case for concern. Where a claim is made by an NHS patient, that money comes from the NHS Budget. Given that it is estimated that around 76% of claims in fact fail, a large proportion of the cost to the NHS may appear to be consumed by legal costs.

A prospect that doctors will base decisions regarding treatment, not on their professional judgement of what is best for their patient but on what is legally safest for the doctor appears very concerning. However, is there any hard evidence that doctors are being forced to practice defensive medicine?

There is the obvious question of what is meant by defensive medicine? In the House of Lords, Lord Pitt argued that "the rising tide of litigation meant that doctors ordered unnecessary and sometimes painful tests, and he predicted an increase in defensive medicine with an alarming waste of resources" (HL Official Report, 10 November, 1987, C 1350-51).

What is undoubtedly true is that many doctors have become alarmed by the growth in malpractice litigation, and how this had damaged the doctor/patient relationship. Doctors in 'highrisks' specialties such as obstetrics and anaesthetics are the worst affected among the medical profession.

Doctors and indeed all health care professionals in England, need to be aware of the reality of the current state of malpractice in the UK. While these claim rates are significant, these are less than in the USA, and awards of compensation are minimal compared to the highest awards in the USA.

However, in the USA, virtually all medical care is provided by the private sector. Most patients carry private health insurance. Their insurer will be as keen as the patient to ensure that any costs arising from medical negligence are recovered from the doctor and his or her insurers. In a private health system such as that operating in the USA, health care is charged on a fee-for-fee basis. The more tests a doctor carries out, the more money he or she makes.

Legal services in the USA are organised on a different basis to those in the UK. Lawyers acting for the clients in negligence actions in the USA, act on a contingency fee basis. If the case fails, the client pays nothing. If the claim succeeds, the lawyer takes a percentage of the damages, normally about one-third.

Such a system makes it much easier for patients to litigate, and gives lawyers a direct interest in the levels of damages awarded. However, English lawyers are now allowed to take on clinical negligence claims on a conditional fee basis.

Solicitors can agree to provide legal service on the basis that they charge no fee if the claim fails, but are permitted to increase their fee by up to 100% if the claim succeeds. However, the claimant remains at risk of having to meet the defendant's legal costs should they lose the case. That significant risk can only be contemplated if the claimant is able to obtain insurance cover against losing their case.

Premiums charged in complex clinical negligence claims can be considerable. Unlike most personal injury claims, those whose income is low enough to qualify may seek legal aid (community legal service funding). However, the majority of adults fall outside that very limited category of eligibility. Also, funding a case of conditional fee arrangements means finding a lawyer who judges a case to be good enough to take it on.

Awards of damages in the USA are decided not by the judge as in the UK, but by the jury. Damages in this country are awarded solely for the purpose of compensating the patient for what they have lost as a result of the defendant doctor's negligence. A US jury is empowered in certain circumstances to double or even treble, compensatory damages by making a further award of punitive damages, to punish the defendant for negligence.

FUNDING A LAWSUIT

Few people are wealthy enough to meet the cost of clinical negligence claims out of their own income or savings. The Access to Justice Act of 1999 removes the former legal aid from most personal injury claims, but remains available in clinical negligence claims.

However, gaining legal aid is not an easy task. Claimants must meet a stringent means test; only adults with a very low income and minimal capital will qualify. Children under 18 are assessed on their own, not their parents' income, so child-patients are still likely to qualify for legal aid.

Even if a potential claimant passes the means test, their case must be strong on its merits. The state will only fund claims likely to succeed. Solicitors able to act for legally-aided clients must be approved by the Legal Service Commission. Only firms which hold a franchise to do legally-aided clinical negligence work can act, and they must be members of a clinical negligence franchise panel.

Conditional fees have become the norm in other personal injury claims. Under a conditional fee agreement (CFA), the solicitor agrees to provide legal services on the basis that unless the claim is successful, the client will pay nothing for the services. If the case is successful, legislation allows the solicitor to charge up to twice the normal fee.

Conditional fees are often styled as 'no win no fee' agreements. The major problems for clinical negligence claimants are two-fold.

Firstly, conditional fees involve risk to the lawyers. They will, obviously, only take on claims if they are satisfied that the majority of the claims on their books will succeed, otherwise the firm will lose money.

Secondly, the no win no fee provision only covers the patient's own solicitor's costs. If the case fails, then the claimant becomes liable for the defendant's hospital or doctor costs also. In most personal injury claims, claimants can buy insurance to cover them against the risk of liability for the defendant's costs. The complexity and expense of clinical negligence claims is such that insurers have been wary about entering this field.

DEFENDING CLAIMS

Until 1990, the medical defence organisations, principally the Medical Defence Union and the Medical Protection Society indemnified individual doctors against personal liability for clinical negligence. Each hospital, health authority or other NHS body met its own costs. The medical defence organisations were powerful players in deciding whether to, and how to defend claims because they paid the doctors' bills.

However, in 1990, NHS Indemnity was introduced to provide hospital trusts indemnity for hospital doctors against liability; while trusts took over the financing and managing of claims. The medical defence organisations continue to meet claims against GPs and claims arising in the private sector.

Then in 1995, the Clinical Negligence Scheme for Trusts (CNST) was established under Section 21 of the NHS and Community Care Act 1990. Membership of the CNST is conditional on trusts complying with risk management procedures. It offers a mutual assurance system so that the individual trust does not run the risk of devastation because of a run of unfortunate losses in the courts complementary to the CNST, the National Health Service Litigation Authority. (NHSLA), is the driving force behind the defence of claims against the NHS today. It exercises significant control over all claims, seeking to ensure swift resolution of indefensible claims and to minimise the cost to the NHS.

Once funding is assured, one of the first practical matters that the patient and their legal advisers must consider is, whom they should sue. The legal doctrine of vicarious liability provides that when a person who is an employee commits a tort in the course of their employment, their employer is also responsible to the victim. The employer will often be better able to pay compensation than an individual employee.

If we look at a claim by a patient who alleges that he suffered injury in the course of treatment as an NHS patient in an NHS hospital, if he can identify a particular individual as negligent, he may proceed against that individual whatever his position in the hospital. In addition, he may also sue that person's employer, which in the case of an NHS trust hospital, this will be the NHS trust itself. Where a hospital doctor is a defendant in the action, payment of any award of compensation made against him is guaranteed because NHS indemnity ensures that any liability incurred by an NHS hospital doctor will be met by his employer. NHS trusts indemnify doctors directly as they have always done for nurses and other hospital employees.

In this case, there is no practical need to bring a claim against the individual doctor. As his or her employer will meet in full any award of compensation, there is little to gain from naming the individual doctor in the claim. However, a doctor who sees his or her reputation on the line, may pressurise his employer to defend the case. As a result, NHS Trusts and the NHSLA may be more prepared to settle the claim swiftly.

There is of course the situation in which suing a doctor individually may be designed not to obtain compensation, but to ensure accountability. The employer to sue, as vicariously liable, in the case of NHS hospital treatment, will normally be the NHS Trust itself.

What is the situation where an NHS patient is treated in a private hospital by virtue of an arrangement between the NHS Trust and a private hospital? What requires examining here is the direct primary liability of the health authority to an NHS patient. The hospital will be liable for any failure of its own. When a patient is admitted for hospital treatment under the NHS, the hospital trust undertakes to provide the patient with reasonably careful, competent and skilled care. Should his or her treatment fall below that standard, the hospital is directly, not just vicariously, responsible to the patient.

Cassidy – v – Minstry of Health, (1951), 2 KB 343.

THE PRIVATE PATIENT

A private patient who engages a private bed in an NHS hospital contracts individually with the surgeon and anaesthetist for the surgery, and the administration of the anaesthetic, and contracts separately with the hospital trust for the nursing and ancillary care. Even if the surgeon and the anaesthetist are employed by the trust when caring for NHS patients, when they act for a private patient, they are acting on their own behalf, and not in the course of their NHS employment. If an error by surgeon or anaesthetist causes the patient injury, he or she can sue only the responsible individual. If the carelessness is that of nursing or other medical staff, he or she may sue the trust.

A patient entering a private hospital needs to consider carefully the nature and scope of their contract. The usual arrangement is similar to that entered into by a private patient taking a private bed within the NHS. The patient engages his own surgeon and anaesthetist who will not be employees of the private hospital. The hospital contracts to provide other medical and nursing care.

Like the private patient within the NHS, the patient must proceed against the surgeon for any error of his, and against the hospital for error by their staff. Some private hospitals and clinics will contract to provide a whole package of care and treatment. When a hospital undertakes to provide total care; the operation, anaesthetic, and post-operative care, and fails to do so, then it is in breach of contract, and liable for its failure to meet the required standard of care.

CLAIMS AGAINST GPs

Most general practitioners are not employees of the NHS. A claim relating to negligence by a GP operating as a single-doctor practice lies against that GP alone. General practices are not covered by NHS Indemnity and are not obliged to belong to a medical defence union. However, the majority of GPs do, but a slight risk remains that a GP sued may be personally uninsured. Where a GP is a member of a partnership, his or her partners may be sued as jointly responsible for any negligence.

If it is not the doctor him or herself who is at fault, but a receptionist or nurse employed by the practice, the GP and his/her partners are vicariously liable as employers. Some difficulty arises in regard to general practices' use of locums and deputising services.

Locums and deputies are not employed by the regular GP practice as a hospital doctor is employed by the NHS. The GP practice is not vicariously liable for every act of negligence on their part. However, a GP practice may be liable for any personal carelessness of its part in selecting a locum or deputising service and failing to check the qualifications of a locum. Also engaging a locum or deputising service without checking whether they carry professional indemnity insurance, may equally constitute a breach of duty to the patient.

WHEN MUST PROCEEDINGS BEGIN?

A patient who is contemplating an action for clinical negligence must act relatively promptly. The general rule is that all actions for personal injuries must be brought within three years of the injury occurring. This is known as the 'limitation period' and is laid down in the Limitation Act 1980. A claim form must be served no later than three years from the date of the alleged negligence.

Sections 11 and 14 of the 1980 Act provide that, where the patient was originally either unaware that he or she has suffered significant injury, or was not aware of the negligence that could have caused their injury, then the three-year period will begin only from the time when they did discover the relevant facts.

All is not quite lost for the patient who delays beyond three years or who is ignorant of the law in this area. A judge may still allow him or her to start an action later. Under Section 33 of the 1980 Act, the court has discretion to override the three-year limitation period, where in all the circumstances, it is fair to all parties to do so.

This three-year limitation period applies only to starting legal proceedings. Once started, action can drag on for years before settlement is agreed. Another important aspect of the rules on limitation is that where the injured patient is under a legal disability at the time that he or she suffers injury, and is under the age of 18 or mentally incapacitated, the limitation period does not begin to run until he or she reaches the age of majority (21) or ceases to be mentally incapacitated.

This means that, for example, a baby might be injured at

birth, and the obstetrician could face an action in respect of the injury up to 21 years after the event. However, the child's parents are free to bring the action earlier on their child's behalf. Parents no longer face a financial deterrent to taking action at the earliest possible stage to obtain compensation for their child. Unlike 1990, previous legal aid rules provided that if they did take action, their income would be taken into account in assessing the child's eligibility for legal aid.

CIVIL JUSTICE REFORM

Cost, complexity and delay were inherent in all actions for compensation, not just clinical negligence cases, in the latter years of the 20th century. Consequently, the civil justice system was perceived as inadequate One of England's most senior judges at this time, Lord Woolf, was commissioned to conduct a review of the civil justice system and to recommend radical reform. He issued his final report in 1996: *Access to Justice: Final Report to the Lord Chancellor on the Civil Justice System in England and Wales*, (HMSO, 1996).

Lord Woolf set out a number of enlightened objectives for the civil justice system. It should be just in its results, the operation of the system should be fair to all parties, costs should be proportionate to the nature of the case. Claims must be dealt with reasonably swiftly. The process should be understandable to all who use it, including any litigant who chooses not to engage a lawyer but to sue in person. There shall be certainty in the way the process works and civil justice should be adequately resourced and reasonably funded.

Four key features of the Woolf reforms are central to medical malpractice litigation. In December 1998, the Pre-Action Protocol for the Resolution of Clinical Disputes was issued. This protocol seeks to fund less adversarial and more cost-effective ways of resolving disputes about health care.

In April, 1999, the Civil Procedure Rules came into force. These rules introduce a united set of procedures for claims, regardless of whether a claim is heard in the County Court or the High Court. Integral to the rules is the concept of care-management. Judges are given infinitely greater powers to manage cases. The rules governing expert witnesses are altered, seeking to abolish the misuse of expert evidence in such actions.

THE CLINICAL NEGLIGENCE PROTOCOL

The protocol establishes what can be described as ground rules for dealing with disputes at their early stages. In essence, it strives to encourage a greater climate of openness between the parties, and recommends a timed sequence of events when disputes do arise.

The protocol's main aim is to restore the relationship between the aggrieved patient and health care professionals and providers. From this approach, it is hoped that disputes can be resolved without recourse to litigation. It is communication between the parties which is the prime objective of the protocol. Full consideration is to be given to early settlement.

Ideally, when a patient believes that they have a case in clinical negligence, in a matter of months they will be able to judge whether their belief is well founded. Also, the defendant doctor or hospital will be in a position to settle any sustainable claims quickly. To this end, the protocol focuses on pre-action events before any claim form has been issued, and the formal stages of litigation begins.

Requests for health records should be met within 40 days of application at a cost no greater than if the patient requested their records under the Data Protection Act, 1998.

The request must provide sufficient information for the doctor or hospital to know if the injury of which the patient complains, is serious, and has serious consequences, and the request must be as specific as possible about which records are required. Just as the potential defendant must not keep the claimant in the dark, so too the protocol aims to ensure that claimants and their lawyers are transparent.

A patient who is considering initiating litigation should send a letter of claim identifying any alleged negligence, their injuries and any consequential financial losses. The letter or claim must identify relevant documents and give sufficient information to enable the defendant to commence investigations and evaluate the claim. The patient may choose to include an offer to settle the case, stating his or her valuation of what would constitute satisfactory compensation. The formal legal proceedings should not be issued until three months after the letter of claim.

The potential defendant must acknowledge the letter of claim within 14 days, and within 3 months must provide a reasoned answer. This letter of response must make it clear if the claim or part of the claim is admitted, and if admissions are binding. If the claim is denied totally, specific answers must be given to the patient's allegations. If additional documents are relied on, these must be disclosed. Where the patient made an offer to settle, the doctor or hospital must respond to that offer. Every opportunity to resolve the case without going to court must be explored.

The protocol also aims to ensure that NHS hospitals and their staff understand the law. It further encourages proper risk assessment, prompt action when adverse outcomes do occur, and good communication with patients. When the protocol works, patients should have no incentive to rush into litigation and both sides should have every incentive to work together. However, what happens if the parties do not cooperate and comply with the protocol? Breaches of the protocol can result in sanctions against both parties and their respective lawyers. Parties may be refused extensions of time to serve claim forms, and costs may be disallowed for unnecessary proceedings.

COMPULSORY DISCLOSURE OF RECORDS

The patient seeking to compel disclosure of records will rely on Section 33 of the Supreme Court Act 1981. He or she can apply for a court order requiring the doctor or hospital whom they plan to sue, to disclose any records or notes likely to be relevant in forthcoming proceedings. Section 34 goes further. The court may order a person who is not a party to the proceedings to produce relevant documents. So, if the patient has started proceedings against a GP or a private medical practitioner, but believes that the hospital or clinic holds notes of value to his or her claim, the hospital or clinic can then be made to disclose the notes. This will help the private patient in a dilemma, as to whether he or she should proceed against doctor or hospital.

Hospitals fear 'fishing expeditions' by aggrieved patients; yet the Clinical Negligence Protocol encourages voluntary disclosure of records. Initially, hospitals preferred to disclose records to the patient's medical adviser alone, and not to the patient or his or her lawyer. In fact, they argued that this was the limit of their obligation.

However, the House of Lords disagreed. The Supreme Court Act of 1981 appears less favourable to patients. It allows terms to be imposed on disclosure by the courts. A court may limit disclosure to (a) the patient's legal advisers, or (b) the patient's legal and medical advisers, or (c) if the patient has no legal adviser, to his medical or other professional adviser. It is up to the court to decide whether the patient sees the records. As long as he or she has retained a lawyer, their lawyer must be permitted to examine the documents.

Three important matters on disclosure need mention here. First, the intention to bring proceedings and the likelihood that they will go ahead, must be real, before the court will order disclosure. The patient must have some solid ground for believing he or she has a claim. They cannot use an application for disclosure to mount a fishing expedition on the off chance that some evidence of negligence will come to light (Dunning v Liverpool Hospital's Board of Governors (1973) 2 All ER 454).

A patient simply wondering if he or she has a claim, but not yet even ready to approach a lawyer, may apply to see their records under the Data Protection Act 1998. This then raises the question: Will the patient be able to see notes of any inquiry ordered by the hospital into their misadventure? The position is complex. If the inquiry was held mainly to provide the basis of information on which legal advice about the authority's legal liability is based, these records are protected by legal professional privilege.

If the main purpose of the inquiry was otherwise, for example, to improve hospital procedures or to provide the basis of disciplinary proceedings against staff, then the patient may be allowed access to the notes of the inquiry (Naylor v Preston Area Health Authority (1987) 2 All ER 353).

The court retains the power to refuse to order disclosure where to do so would be injurious to the public interest. However, this is very unlikely to be the case where what is asked for is the patient's own medical notes.

CASE MANAGEMENT

If attempts to resolve a claim fail, and the patient commences formal proceedings, the conduct of the case will be strictly controlled. There will be an emphasis on enforcing time limits and keeping costs down. The claim will be allocated a track. A clinical negligence claim that was worth less than £1,000 would theoretically be allocated to the small claims track. Such claims will usually be resolved within the established complaints procedures. Claims worth between £1,000 and £ 15,000 are allocated to the fast track. This means that the case should be resolved within a period of 30 weeks. The actual court hearing should take no more than one day, and oral expert evidence is limited. Claims worth more than £15,000 or where the issues are especially complex, these go on to the multi-track, where judges control the allocation process. Most clinical negligence claims will be multi-track.

PROVING NEGLIGENCE: THE ROLE OF THE EXPERT

How does the patient prove negligence? The onus lies on him or her. The patient must demonstrate that it is more likely than not, that his or her deterioration in health or their injury resulted from the negligence of the defendant. How does the claimant discharge the onus of proof? In the majority of cases, he or she will be reliant on expert testimony.

They will need to put forward medical evidence to demonstrate two vital factors. Firstly, that there was negligence, on the part of the defendant, or a person for whom the defendant was responsible. Secondly, that the relevant negligence caused the harm of which he or she complains.

The Civil Procedure Rules of 1998 state that the expert's primary duty is to the court in matters involving their expertise. This duty overrides any obligation to the person from whom instructions were received, or by whom the expert receives payment. These rules also impose limits on the use of expert evidence or testimony. To this end, expert testimony must be restricted to what is reasonably required to resolve a particular case. In addition, the court has power to direct the appointment of a single joint expert rather than each party choosing their own experts. Obviously, if a single expert is to be appointed, it makes sense for the parties themselves to agree on this single expert. Such cases will be rare and limited to cases where there is no substantial medical dispute regarding causation or prognosis.

The majority of clinical negligence cases will involve disputes about establishing whether there was any negligence in the first place, whether the negligence caused the injuries of which the claimant complains, and what the likely prognosis.

Such issues may well require separate expert testimony. If there is no complexity regarding causation, a single expert should be agreed to address particular issues. As much of the expert evidence as possible should be in writing, oral testimony is allowable only with the permission of the court.

Where there are multiple experts, all correspondence, documents and instructions must be disclosed to the experts, and there must be multiple disclosure of all expert's reports. This is to ensure transparency in the proceedings.

Meetings of experts are encouraged to resolve the differences between them, and possibly promote resolution of the case without proceeding to an actual court hearing. It is now common practice that the parties' lawyers may be present at meetings of experts.

WHEN THE BURDEN OF PROOF SHIFTS TO THE DOCTOR

In the majority of cases, the patient must prove negligence and the doctor is not called on to prove his or her innocence. However, there is a general rule of the law of negligence, that where the defendant is in complete control of the relevant events, and then an accident occurs, that could have been avoided if proper care had been taken, then the fact that the accident did occur, affords reasonable evidence of negligence.

The defendant will be held liable unless he or she can advance an explanation of the accident which is consistent with the exercise of proper care by him or her. This rule is generally known as 'res ipsa loquitur' from the Latin meaning 'the thing speaks for itself'.

This rule can be applied to clinical negligence cases, but the courts are reluctant to do so.

Initially, it was argued that the rule applied only where everyone of reasonable intelligence would know that accidents of a certain nature do not ordinarily happen without negligence.

However, since most people are not medically qualified, they would have great difficulty in knowing whether the accident was one which could or could not happen if proper care was taken. The Court of Appeal said that expert medical evidence was admissible to establish what should or should not occur if ordinary care was exercised (Mahon v Osborne (1939) 2 KB 14). For example, sometimes after an abdominal surgical operation, a swab or even a pair of forceps is discovered in the patient's body. Without evidence of a quite exceptional nature, it is very clear that someone has been careless.

Res ipsa is also of value to the NHS patient who has undoubtedly suffered because someone was negligent either in the operating theatre or in the course of post-operative care, but the patient cannot identify that particular person. If every member of the staff who might be responsible is employed by the hospital, then an inference of negligence is raised against the hospital, who are vicariously liable for whoever the culprit may be (Roe v Ministry of Health (1954) 2 QB 66).

AWARDS OF COMPENSATION

Once a patient has satisfied the court that there has been negligence by the defendant as a result of which he or she suffered harm, what damages can they expect to receive?

There are no special rules governing clinical negligence awards. The patient's damages will be assessed to compensate him or her for any actual or prospective loss of earnings, and for the pain, suffering and disability that they have endured and will endure. Their compensation for loss of earnings will indicate a sum representing any period in which they would, if not for the injury, have expected to be alive and earning. Additional to these sums to represent what he or she has lost, the patient will be awarded an amount to cover extra expenses that he or she and family will incur.

However, the patient must usually sue within three years. At that stage, a prognosis about future health is speculative. Under Section 32A of the Supreme Court Act 1981, the court has power to make an award of provisional damages based on the assumption that the prospect of further damage or deterioration will not materialise. Should it do so at some later date, the patient may return to court to request a further award to compensate them for the consequences of that damage or deterioration.

With the exception of Section 32A of the 1981 Act, unless the parties agree to set up a structured settlement, damages have to be assessed on a once and forever basis as a lump sum. Courts will seek to ensure that the sum awarded is such as will be wholly exhausted by care of the patient, with no surplus left over as a bonus for relatives.

An anomaly in the law is that the claimant may be able to claim for the full cost of any private medical care he or she selects regardless of whether such facilities are available free on the NHS. This raises an obvious question; what happens if the defendant argues that the claimant could have avoided serious disability and consequent loss of income?

For example, a patient is injured by a negligently performed spinal operation. Doctors recommend corrective surgery but the patient refuses to agree and is left unable to work. The Privy Council makes it clear that a court should only reduce the compensation payable to the patient for his or her disability if the defendant hospital can prove that the decision to refuse surgery was unreasonable.

Changes in the law relating to damages have contributed to the increase in compensation payable in negligence claims against the NHS. Awards of over £3 million are not that uncommon today. Improved medical skills mean that patients who suffer injury as a consequence of medical mistakes live much longer. Greater opportunities exist to improve their quality of life. When negligence results in a patient's death, compensation for the bereavement occasioned to their family is only available to parents of children under 18, or to spouses. The level of compensation was set at £10,000 in 2002. For example, should a patient be left paralysed from the waist down by an anaesthetist's mistake, the defendant hospital will have to cover the cost of future care and equipment.

STRUCTURED SETTLEMENTS

Some of the uncertainties generated by having to assess compensation as a lump sum, are avoidable by resort to Structure Settlements. The settlement is devised to meet the actual needs of the patient over time. He or she will receive an initial capital sum to cover actual losses already quantified and such matters as compensation for pain and suffering. The remainder of the money will be used by the defendant to purchase an annuity for the claimant's benefit. The annuity will be flexible to adapt to the changing circumstances of the patient. The income received by the patient is not taxable. Should he or she die earlier than anticipated, payments cease.

In an ordinary personal injury claim, the defendant's insurers arrange the settlement and negotiate the purchase of annuities. NHS structured settlements are usually self-financed. They use their own income to arrange periodic payments building the settlement into budgets. Tax concessions aid this process. Structured settlements in large claims save the NHS money. However, not all claimants agree to such a settlement. Distrust may cause them to be suspicious or want more control over the investment of their own money.

CHAPTER SIX:
Case Studies

In this final chapter, the reader is presented with three case studies, each concerned with a specific aspect of clinical negligence, and all of which have been discussed in detail in the text.

The first case centres upon the issue of blood transfusions to a patient who was a practising Jehovah's Witness. It is concerned with the anticipatory refusal of consent in which the patient is unconscious and whose life is in danger. It highlights the undue influence of the patient's mother's religious beliefs. This case also emphasises the hospital and doctors' duty when in doubt about a patient's consent, to resort to the necessity principle in such situations.

The second case is concerned with failure to act within clinical negligence actions. The patient in this case suffered a cerebral stroke as a result of dangerously high blood pressure. The claimant's action centred upon whether the period between the consultant's consultations with his patient had been too long, and were, therefore, negligent.

This case questions whether it was negligent on the consultant's part not to have acted much earlier in response to ambulatory blood pressure monitoring results. This, the claimant claimed, would have avoided the patient suffering a second haemorrhage, resulting in paralysis.

The final case is concerned with a doctor's failure to warn his patient of the risks in consenting to an operation. In fact, the patient suffered injury when the anticipatory risk actually materialised during the course of surgery. The action by the claimant sought to establish that she would not have undergone the recommended operation if she had been 'properly' advised by the surgeon. The case established that the causation aspect of the action had been established by the claimant, and that the consultant's failure to warn was sufficient to establish causation in such cases.

CASE ONE

RE: T (ADULT: REFUSAL OF MEDICAL TREATMENT

COURT OF APPEAL: CIVIL DIVISION

Lord Donaldson of Lymington MR; Butler-Sloss and Staughton, LJJ

JULY, 1992

Council for T: James Munby QC and Christopher Butler.
Council for Two Health Authorities: David Stembridge QC and Stephen Oliver-Jones.
Counsel for T's Father: Allan Levy QC and Peter Rank.
Council for T's Mother: Richard Daniel.

CASE SUMMARY

On 4 July 1992, Miss T, who was 20 years old and 34 weeks pregnant, was admitted to hospital. Pneumonia was diagnosed and the narcotic drug Pethidine was administered, along with antibiotics. Miss T, though not herself a practising Jehovah's Witness, had been brought up in that faith by her mother who was. On 5 July, Miss T was receiving oxygen and further doses of Pethidine; she was heavily sedated and in great pain. Following a visit from her mother during which they were alone together, Miss T announced out of the blue that, because of her religious beliefs, she did not want a blood transfusion. She repeated her objection to Dr F immediately afterwards. When Miss T indicated her belief that there were alternatives to blood transfusions, Dr F assured her that transfusions were often not necessary after a caesarean delivery. Miss T thereafter signed a form, which was neither read nor explained to her, indicating her refusal of consent to blood transfusions. Early on 6 July, Miss T was delivered of a stillborn baby by caesarean section. Her condition deteriorated and that night she was transferred to the intensive care unit. An abscess developed on Miss T's lungs which indicated the need for a blood transfusion, but because of her expressed wishes, the consultant felt inhibited from administering one. Miss T was put on a ventilator and received paralysing drugs. Throughout 7 July she remained sedated and in a critical condition.

Miss T's father sought a declaration from Ward, J, that it would not be unlawful for the hospital to administer a blood transfusion to Miss T notwithstanding her absence of consent. After taking evidence by telephone from Doctor F, that Miss T had not been fully 'compos mentis' or rational when she signed the form refusing consent, Ward J, granted an interlocutory declaration at 1.30am on 9 July. Miss T immediately received a transfusion of blood or plasma. At a full hearing before Ward, J, on 10 July, Dr F changed his evidence completely. Ward J, held (1) that Miss T had been mentally competent and had the capacity to decide for herself, notwithstanding the influence of Pethidine and of pain upon her; (2) Miss T made her decision under the influence of her mother but this did not constitute undue influence and did not vitiate her consent; (3) taking into account the depth of Miss T's religious convictions and the circumstances in which she announced her decision, her refusal of a blood transfusion did not cover the emergency which had arisen which had been outside her contemplation and that of others. Ward J, issued a further declaration on the terms of that of 9 July. The Official Solicitor, acting as 'guardian ad litem' of Miss T, who was unconscious, appealed against the declaration of Ward J.

HELD

(1) There was no valid refusal of consent to blood transfusion by Miss T and the administering of a blood transfusion was justified by the 'Principle of Necessity'. The appeal would therefore by dismissed.
(2) A competent patient's right of choice existed whether the reasons for making the choice are irrational, unknown or non-existent. Miss T had been subjected to the undue influence of her mother which vitiated her consent.

LORD DONALDSON MR

This appeal has a wider purpose, namely to give guidance to hospital authorities and to the medical profession in situations involving a refusal to consent to treatment. A patient's interest consists of his right to self determination. Society's interest is in upholding the concept that all human life is sacred and should be preserved if possible. In a situation where these two interests conflict, the right of the individual is paramount. But where there is doubt, the doubt falls to be resolved in favour of the preservation of life. The next of kin of a patient incompetent to consent, has no legal rights either to consent or to refuse consent to treatment.

However, providing the interests of the patient are not adversely affected by any consequential delay, contacting the next of kin may reveal that the patient has made an anticipatory choice which, if clearly established and applicable in the circumstances, would bind the medical practitioner. But neither the personal circumstances of the patient, nor speculation as to what the patient would have chosen, can bind a practitioner in his or her choice of whether, or not, to treat. Nor would it justify him in acting contrary to a clearly established anticipatory refusal to accept treatment. However, there are factors to be taken into account in determining what treatment is in the best interests of the patient. When considering the effect of a decision made by a previously competent patient, now incompetent, doctors should consider the scope and basis of that decision. They cannot conclude that had the patient the capacity to do so, he or she would reverse their decision in the changed situation.

A refusal of treatment ceases to be effective if the changed factual situation falls outside the scope of the refusal, or if the assumption on which it is based is false. Doctors then face a situation in which no decision has been made and have the right and the duty to treat the patient in his or her best interests. Where there is doubt about the validity of a patient's refusal of essential treatment, doctors or hospital authorities should at once seek a declaration from the courts, as to the lawfulness of the proposed treatment. At the conclusion of the argument, their Lordship stated that they would file their decision on 24 July, 1992, and their reasons thereafter on a later date. The court announced that the appeal would be dismissed.

SUMMARY OF THE JUDGEMENT

Miss T's Case History

On Wednesday, 1 July 1992, when Miss T was 34 weeks pregnant, she was involved in a road traffic accident. She went to hospital where she complained of pains in her right shoulder and in the right side of her chest. She was not initially X-rayed because of her pregnant condition, but was advised to rest and to take an analgesic. She returned to the hospital in the early hours of Saturday, 4 July complaining of increased chest pains. She was X-rayed and diagnosed as suffering from pleurisy or pneumonia. She was prescribed antibiotics and analgesics including Pethidine which is a narcotic drug, and also given oxygen. It is at this point that timings become important. The hospital's patient assessment form contains the entry: "Religious belief and relevant practices: Jehovah's Witness (ex) but still has certain beliefs and practices".

Miss T was admitted to the Ward at 6.10am and given 50mg of Pethidine, together with antibiotics at 6.55am. At that time, she was very breathless and complaining of severe chest and shoulder pains. Later during the morning, she had a lung scan which did not reveal any abscess but showed a picture which was consistent with pneumonia. No alteration was made in her treatment. Shortly after 1.00pm Miss T was given another dose of Pethidine. At 6.30pm Miss T's mother arrived at the hospital accompanied by C. Later that night, according to information given by the hospital to Miss T's father, Miss T received more Pethidine. Miss T's father arrived at the hospital at 8.30am on Sunday 5 July. He observed that his daughter was heavily sedated, and that her breathing was extremely laboured. The nursing staff told her father that she had no rest during the night and was in considerable pain. She was receiving oxygen and had to be raised every 30 minutes to enable her to clear sputum from her lungs, a process with which the father assisted.

Miss T's father was anxious as to any complications which might arise from her mother's religious beliefs and spoke to a doctor whom he was unable later to identify. He was told that Miss T did not require a blood transfusion and that there was no need for concern. The situation would be resolved if a transfusion were required. He also noticed a reduction in Miss T's awareness of what was going on around her and mentioned this to the nursing staff, who told him it was the effect of the drugs. During Sunday morning, Miss T's father became so concerned with her apparent condition that he telephoned his mother (the paternal grandmother), who arrived at 11am. At 2.50pm, Miss T received the last dose of Pethidine before 5pm when she, for the first time, spoke of the possibility of a blood transfusion. Meanwhile, C and Miss T's sister arrived at the hospital, as did Miss T's mother. Miss T's mother and father had an argument, but not in the presence of Miss T, and agreed that they would not allow their acrimonious relationship come to her notice. The evidence does not reveal whether this argument was about or involved the topic of blood transfusions.

For some time before 5pm, her mother was alone with Miss T. What passed between them we do not know, and the mother, although a party to the proceedings, has never seen fit to give evidence. At 5pm, a staff nurse joined Miss T and her mother, and Miss T told the staff nurse that she did not want a blood transfusion, that she used to be a Jehovah's Witness and that she still maintained some beliefs. The staff nurse said that she thought it strange that this statement should have been volunteered 'out of the blue', moments after her mother had arrived. However, she thought that at that stage Miss T was able to understand what was going on. She sought to 'pacify' Miss T and did not think that there was any problem as Miss T did not need a blood transfusion. At 7.30pm Miss T's father returned to the ward and thought that her condition was worsening and that she appeared disorientated.

Shortly afterwards, Miss T went into labour and at 10.45pm a decision was reached that she should be transferred to the maternity unit. This involved conveyance in an ambulance for some 200 to 300 yards, during which time Miss T was again alone with her mother. They arrived at the unit about 11.30pm. Miss T was then examined by the obstetrics registrar who found her to be in a distressed condition with respiratory pain and contractions. A decision was made that the delivery should be by Caesarean section. Shortly afterwards, Miss T told the midwife that she did not want a blood transfusion. Immediately afterwards, Dr F saw Miss T and said: "Do you object to blood transfusions?" She replied: "Yes". Dr F said: "Does that mean that you do not want a blood transfusion?" Miss T replied: "No". Afterwards, Miss T said: "You can use other things though, can't you, like sugar solutions?" Dr F said that he cannot remember the exact conversation which followed but: "I said that we could use other solutions to expand the blood, but they were not as effective as blood at transporting oxygen. I also tried to reassure Miss T and her father than blood transfusions were not often necessary after a Caesarean section".

As Dr F was leaving, the midwife produced a form of refusal of consent to blood transfusion which Miss T signed and the midwife countersigned. The form contemplated that it would be also countersigned by an obstetrician but it was not so signed. Contrary to what was stated on the form, it was not explained to Miss T that it may be necessary to give a blood transfusion so as to prevent injury to her health or even to preserve life, nor was the form read or its contents explained to her. She simply signed blindly. Although C had no recollection of the fact, it was found that he was present at the same time when Miss T was expressing her wish not to have a blood transfusion. The Caesarean section was performed in the early hours of Monday 6 July, but unfortunately the baby was stillborn.

The same night Miss T's condition deteriorated and she was transferred to the intensive care unit. It appears that although there had previously been no abscess in Miss T's lungs, one had developed. The situation as it then existed was such that, given a free hand, the consultant anaesthetist in charge of the unit, would unhesitantly have administered a blood transfusion, but felt inhibited from doing so in the light of Miss T's expressed wishes. Miss T was put on a ventilator and paralysing drugs were administered. She remained sedated and in a critical condition throughout Tuesday, 7 July, although she showed some slight improvement. On Wednesday 8 July, Miss T's father and C decided to seek the assistance of the court. It was one which, in all the circumstances, should have been taken by the hospital authority themselves on the Monday.

Their request for assistance was referred to a circuit judge Ward J, which was about 3pm. He made immediate inquiries by telephone, but felt that there was insufficient evidence to justify his intention. However, he did think the situation was grave enough to justify further investigation. Mt Alan Levy QC, who had extensive experience of cases of this type was consulted. As a result, Mr Levy, his junior counsel and their instructing solicitors, together with Miss T's father and C, attended at the judge's lodgings shortly after 11pm that same evening. Ward J, took evidence on the telephone from Dr F, who had spoken to Miss T in the maternity unit after she had stated for the second time, that she did not wish to have a blood transfusion and before she had signed the refusal form.

WARD J. JUDGMENT

"Dr F told me in summary that (Miss T) was under the influence of the narcotic drug Pethidine. Her demeanour late on that Sunday evening was drowsy and detached. He expressed the opinion that she was not fully compos mentis, that she was not fully rational in making an assessment of her medical condition being unaware how critical her condition was, and that she was not fully rational at the time of signing the refusal. In those circumstances, I considered (at 1.30am) that I had no option but to grant the interlocutory relief that was sought by way of a declaration that in the circumstances which were then prevailing, it would not be unlawful for the hospital to administer a blood transfusion to Miss T, despite the absence of her consent because that appeared manifestly to be in her best interests."

The matter again came before Ward J, on Friday 10 July for a full hearing, at which he heard evidence from the doctors and nurses involved. In essence, Ward J, found that the physical and mental state of Miss T on the Sunday afternoon and evening, were such that although she was undoubtedly under the influence of her mother, she was capable of reaching, and did reach a decision as to her own treatment. However, he went on to find that Miss T was lulled into a sense of false security by hospital staff, and that she was misinformed as to the availability and effectiveness of alternative procedures. Against this background and his assessment of the shallowness of Miss T's acceptance of the beliefs of the Jehovah's Witnesses, he considered Miss T's refusal of treatment by blood transfusion as not extending to the question of whether or not she should receive transfusions in the extreme situation which had arisen. In other words, he concluded that, Miss T had never consented nor refused. As Miss T was no longer able to express any view, it was a classic emergency situation in which it was lawful for the doctors to treat her in whatever way they considered to be in her best interests.

THE HEARING AT THE COURT OF APPEAL

Lord Donaldson's Summing-Up

"For the strictly limited purpose of deciding whether Ward J's decision should be affirmed or reversed, it suffices to say that an appellate court should always be slow to reject a trial judge's findings of fact, he having had the advantage of seeing and hearing the witnesses. On that basis, I would be content to say, as we did say at the conclusion of this hearing, that the appeal should be dismissed, and that we affirm Ward J's declaration that it would be lawful for the hospital to administer blood to Miss T. However, this appeal has a wider purpose, namely to give guidance to hospital authorities and to the medical profession, on the appropriate response to a refusal by an adult to accept treatment. The fact that 'emergency cases' apart, no medical treatment of an adult patient of full capacity can be undertaken without his consent, creates a situation in which the absence of consent has much the same effect as a refusal. That does not necessarily create any problem for doctors or hospitals. On some occasions it may not be of great importance to the patient's health whether he is treated at the time or perhaps at all, or it may be a question of choices. The doctor may advise that treatment A is preferable to treatment B, but that he is prepared to undertake either.

The patient may elect for and consent to treatment B, thereby declining consent to treatment A. Where the problem arises in the comparatively rare situations in which an adult patient declines to consent to treatment which in the clinical judgment of those attending him is necessary if irreparable damage is not to be done to his health or, in the same cases, if his life is to be saved. It is only in that context that this appeal may afford guidance to the doctors and hospitals. Doctors faced with a refusal of consent have to give very careful and detailed consideration to the patient's capacity to decide at the time when the decision was made. It may not be the simple case of the patient having no capacity because, for example, at that time he had hallucinations. It may be the more difficult case of a temporarily reduced capacity at the time when the decision was made. What matters is that the doctors should consider whether at that time, he had a capacity which was commensurate with the gravity of the situation which he purported to make. The more serious the decision, the greater the capacity required. If the patient had the requisite capacity, they are bound by his decision. If not, they are free to treat him in what they believe to be in his best interests.

This problem is more likely to arise at a time when the patient is unconscious and cannot be consulted. If he can be consulted, this should be done, but again full account has to be taken of his then capacity to make up his own mind. A special problem may arise if at the time the decision is made, the patient has been subjected to the influence of some third party. This is by no means to say that the patient is not entitled to receive and indeed invite advice and assistance from others in reaching a decision, particularly from members of his family. But the doctors have to consider whether the decision is really that of the patient. It is wholly acceptable that the patient should have been persuaded by others of the merits of such a decision and have decided accordingly. It matters not how strong the persuasion was, so long as it did not overbear the independence of the patient's decision. The real question in each such case is, does the patient really mean what he says or is he merely saying it for a quiet life, to satisfy someone else or because the advice and persuasion to which he has been subjected is such that he can no longer think and decide for himself?

When considering the effect of outside influences, two aspects can be of crucial importance. First, the strength of the will of the patient. One who is very tired, in pain or depressed, will be much less able to resist having his will overborne than one who is rested; free from pain and relatively positive in outlook. Second, relationship of the 'persuader' to the patient may be of crucial importance. Persuasion based upon religious belief can also be much more compelling and the fact that arguments based upon religious beliefs are being deployed by someone in a very close relationship with the patient, will give them added force, and should alert the doctors to the possibility that the patient's capacity or will to decide has been overborne.

CONCLUDING SUMMARY

(1) Prima facie every adult has the right and capacity to decide whether or not he or she will accept medical treatment even if a refusal may risk permanent injury to his or her health or even lead to premature death. However, the

presumption of capacity to decide which stems from the fact that the patient is an adult, is rebuttable.

(2) An adult patient may be deprived of his or her capacity to decide either by long-term mental incapacity or retarded development, or by temporary factors such as unconsciousness or confusion, or the effects of fatigue, shock, pain or drugs.

(3) If an adult patient did not have the capacity to decide at the time of the purported refusal and still does not have the capacity to decide at the time of the purported refusal and still does not have the capacity, it is the duty of the doctors to treat him or her in whatever way they consider in the exercise of their clinical judgment, to be in his or her best interests.

(4) Doctors faced with a refusal of consent have to give very careful and detailed consideration to what the patient's capacity to decide at the time when the decision was made. It may be a case of reduced capacity. What matters is whether at that time, the patient's capacity was reduced below the level needed in the case of a refusal of that importance.

(5) In some cases, doctors will not only have to consider the capacity of the patient to refuse treatment, but also whether the refusal has been vitiated because it resulted not from the patient's will, but from the will of others. It matters not that those others sought, however strongly, to persuade the patient to refuse, so long as in the end, the refusal represented the patient's independent decision. If, however, his or her will was overborne, the refusal will not have represented a true decision. In this context, the relationship of the persuader to the patient, for example, spouse, parents or religious adviser, will be important.

(6) In all cases, doctors will need to consider what is the true scope and basis of the refusal. Was it intended to apply in the circumstances which have arisen? Was it based upon assumptions which in the event have not been realised?

(7) Forms of Refusal should be designed to bring the consequences of a refusal forcibly to the attention of patients.

(8) In cases of doubt, as to the effect of a purported refusal of treatment, where failure to treat threatens the patient's life or threatens irreparable damage to his or her health, doctors and health authorities should not hesitate to apply to the courts for assistance.

Source: Butterworths Medico-Legal Reports: (9 BMLR (1992) pp 46-68).

CASE TWO

LOWE v HAVERING HOSPITAL NHS TRUST

THE HIGH COURT OF JUSTICE – QUEEN'S BENCH DIVISION

Judge Peter Crawford, QC

JUNE, 2001

Counsel for the Claimant: David Wilby QC and Henry Charles.
Counsel for the Defendant: Andrew Collender QC and Anna Garratt.

CASE SUMMARY

In April, 1995, the claimant Mr Leonard Henry Lowe aged 36 at the time, suffered a cerebral stroke of mild to moderate severity. It was discovered that he suffered from chronic hypertension (high blood pressure). He was referred to Dr Pearson, employed at one of the hospitals managed by the defendant trust, as a consultant physician specialising in clinical pharmacology. Dr Pearson saw the claimant four times over a four-week period from 27 September 1995. Then after a gap of two months, a fifth consultation took place followed by a sixth consultation on 24 January, 1996. In between the fifth and sixth consultations, the claimant's blood pressure was measured continuously over 24 hours from 4/5 January 1996. These recordings showed readings of 172 and 116, and 199 over 145. All the expert witnesses agreed that those readings were dangerously high. However, Dr Pearson did not consider those readings required him to see the claimant earlier than the scheduled appointment on 24 January 1996.

On that day, Dr Pearson modified slightly the claimant's medication.

The following day (25 January, 1996), the claimant suffered a second stroke, much more damaging than the first, which left him permanently and severely disabled, with severe speech problems, rendering him almost incomprehensible. The action for damages alleged negligence by Dr Pearson in:

- Failing to analyse the ambulatory blood pressure readings of 4/5 January until or close to 24 January, and to take more urgent action based on these readings.
- Failing to institute a proper and sufficient regime of treatment following the consultation on 24 January.
- Failing to arrange for the claimant's blood pressure to be monitored at a review between the dates of the fifth and sixth consultations.

It was held that there were four issues for the court to consider. Firstly, was the claimant's condition merely hypertension? The court held that the claimant's blood pressure had been dangerously high and unstable. Secondly, what was the risk? In dealing with a risk there are three elements to be taken into account; the likelihood of the risked event actually occurring, the nature of the consequences if the risk did occur, and the degree of ease or difficulty in reducing the likelihood of preventing the risk from occurring. What was the proper medical practice in discharge of the doctor's duty of care? Was the eight-week period between the fifth and sixth consultations a reasonable exercise by Dr Pearson of his skill as a physician? Finally, was proper medical practice observed by the doctor on 24 January 1996?

Two professors giving expert witness testimony for the claimant, were clear and uncompromising in their view that Dr Pearson had failed to comply with a proper standard of care. The expert witnesses for the defence had failed to make sufficient allowance for various special aspects of the claimant's condition.

First, the claimant had not merely a high blood pressure, but an uncontrolled one. Secondly, Dr Pearson had suspicions that the claimant had not been fully compliant with the medication prescribed for him, and that underlined the necessity of seeing the claimant at shorter intervals than might otherwise have been the appropriate. Thirdly, that the claimant was a relatively young man who had a wife and a dependant family.

These were things which a physician should properly have taken into account in his general care of the patient. It was plain that Dr Pearson had given these factors no particular consideration. In fixing a two-month period of review and in not acting on the results of the ambulatory reading more swiftly, Dr Pearson had breached his duty of care to the claimant.

On the issue of causation, the court accepted the evidence of the claimant's experts that if the claimant's medication had been changed as late as early January 1996, the risk of the second stroke would have been reduced by at least 50%. The two breaches of care by Dr Pearson, had been causative of the claimant's loss, and he was therefore, liable. Leonard Lowe sought damages in an action for negligence against the defendant hospital trust based on an absence of proper and adequate medical care when he was referred to a consultant physician for chronic hypertension, which resulted in the claimant suffering a second cerebral stroke.

THE CASE HISTORY

The claimant, Mr Leonard Henry Lowe was born on 30 June, 1958 and in 2001 was almost 43 years of age. On 13 April, 1995, the claimant suffered a bleed on the brain, which constituted a cerebral stroke. It was a stroke of mild to moderate severity; he was taken to hospital, where he was examined. It was discovered that he suffered from chronic hypertension, his blood pressure was too high. It had probably been too high for a long time and it manifested itself on that occasion by a bleed on the brain. He was treated at the Oldchurch and Harold Wood Hospitals NHS Trust, both of them part of the Havering Hospitals NHS Trust, the defendants in this action. The claimant's blood pressure was unstable. It was difficult to control and various drugs were tried. Simultaneously, he was undergoing rehabilitation from the effects of the stroke. He made a good recovery which was not entirely complete but substantial.

Because of the instability of the claimant's blood pressure, he was referred to Dr Pearson, who was a member of the defendant's medical staff. It was he who was the specialist responsible for treating hypertensive patients at the defendant's hospitals. The claimant saw Dr Pearson on a number of occasions after he had been referred to him by another doctor at the hospital. The first consultation is recorded on 27 September, 1995, when Dr Pearson saw Mr Lowe, the claimant, in the ward at the hospital. His blood pressure was high, his speech was, to a degree slurred, and Dr Pearson recorded that his findings were showing Grade 3 hypertensive damage. A diagnosis of high blood pressure was obvious and various drugs were prescribed. Following the first consultation, Dr Pearson saw Mr Lowe again on 4 October 1995, on 18 October and then on 25 October, four times within the first month. There was then a gap of one month between the fourth and fifth consultations. Then Dr Pearson saw Mr Lowe on 29 November 1995. On that occasion, his blood pressure was recorded as 150 over 105, and 160 over 110. This was followed by a two-month gap before the next appointment. The profile was four appointments in the first month from 27 September to 25 October, 1995.

This was followed by a gap of one month between the fourth and fifth, then another gap of two months between the fifth and sixth consultation which was arranged for 24 January, 1996. It was during this gap between the fifth and sixth appointments that Dr Pearson arranged for a 24-hour blood pressure recording. Although this was arranged at the consultation on 29 November 1995, it was not instituted until the 4/5 January, 1996. When the recording was made, it showed what all the expert witnesses agreed were dangerously high readings of 172 over 116, and 199 over 145.

It was Dr Pearson's view that those readings while unsatisfactory, did not require earlier intervention, than the appointment arranged for 24 January, 1996. It was the claimant's case, supported by his expert witnesses, that the period from 29 November 1995 to 4/5 January 1996 was too long to comply with the requirements of good practice. Also, that the readings, when they were obtained, indicated a necessity for urgent rather than routine intervention.

It was on these issues that the proceedings turned. Dr Pearson saw Mr Lowe on 24 January 1996, and modified the dose of medication slightly. The next day (25 January) Mr Lowe suffered from a further stroke. This second stroke left him permanently and severely disabled, and this is the foundation for his claim for damages in the action. The consequences of the second stroke are that Mr Lowe is very substantially disabled, has great difficulty in speech, and he is almost entirely immobile.

PLEADINGS

The claimant's claim which was served on the defendants on 18 October 1999, alleged that the defendants failed to analyse the 24-hour ambulatory blood pressure monitoring results received at the hospital on 5 January, 1996 until just before 24 January, 1996. The claim asserts that this potentially dangerous level should have resulted in more urgent action It also alleges that when Dr Pearson knew that the claimant's blood pressure was 180 over 110 on 24

January 1996, he failed to institute a proper and sufficient regime of treatment. It is also alleged that the defendants failed to arrange for the claimant's blood pressure to be monitored at a review between 29 November 1995 and 24 January 1996.

The defendants, in their defence, asserted that the review date for monitoring his blood pressure (24 January 1996) was set for eight weeks after the consultation on 29 November 1995. There was a long waiting list at the material time for 24-hour ambulatory blood readings to be carried out. They also maintained that, in keeping with other NHS hospitals, there was a two-to-three-week gap between recording and forwarding results. However, no evidence was called on behalf of the defendants to support this claim.

ISSUES

(1) What was the nature of the claimant's condition? Was it merely hypertension? A good deal of time was occupied by the medical witnesses in debating this very point during the course of the court hearing. It was accepted on all sides, first, that at all material times, the claimant's blood pressure was high to very high. Second, that it was unstable, and third, the combination of pressure and instability rendered it dangerous.

(2) What was the risk? One view suggested that the risk was relatively low, around 2 or 3 per 100. In another sense, it was high. In dealing with any risk, there are three elements to take into account. The first is the likelihood of the event itself occurring. The second is the nature of the consequences should the event occur. The third is the degree of ease or difficulty in reducing the likelihood of the event occurring.

(3) What was the proper medical practice in discharging the practitioner's duty of care? Did the 8-week gap between 29 November, 1995 and 24 January, 1996 represent a

reasonable exercise by Dr Pearson of his professional skill as a physician? Or was it, as the claimant's witnesses contended, an excessive period in the circumstances?
(4) Was the proper medical practice observed? It was not asserted on behalf of the defendants that Dr Pearson's treatment of this patient was best practice or even good practice according to the defendant's experts. What they did say was that it was acceptable practice, which might have reasonably been followed by a responsible practitioner.

THE EXPERTS

For the claimant were Professor Vallance and Professor O'Grady, for the defendants were Dr Thomas and Professor Brown. There were all medical men of considerable reputation, occupying senior academic and/or consultant posts in the National Health Service. Professors Vallance and O'Grady thought that the interval of two months, from 29 November before the next appointment, was negligently too long. Also, that the failure to act more promptly on the results of the ambulatory review when it was received, was negligently slow. Professor Brown and Dr Thomas thought that, where the first period, indeed both periods, were long and slow, and did not accord with best practice, but that they did accord with acceptable practice.

BREACH OF DUTY

There was a substantial measure of agreement between the experts. This was found in the report of the expert's meeting held on 24, March, 2001. This was attended by both experts for the claimant and defendants. A crucial question on the agenda for this meeting was: "Was the management of the claimant by medication including the adjustments to that medication made by Dr Pearson on 29 November, 1995, acceptable? If it was not acceptable, in what respects did such management fall below an acceptable standard?" According to the judge, the answer was this; alteration in the timing of the medication on the 29 November 1995, was unlikely to have made any difference to Mr Lowe's hypertension. Although there was documentary evidence of raised blood pressure from obtaining the recordings on the 24-hour tape, if there was any doubt about the true level of Mr Lowe's blood pressure, then not altering the hypertensive medication was a reasonable action; this would allow repeated observations of the blood pressure. It appears that the 24-hour ambulatory blood pressure monitoring was requested in order to do this. This action needed to be accompanied by a timely review. It was agreed that although the standard of practice was not ideal, the intended review interval of 8 weeks with an interim recording of blood pressure would reflect, and be consistent with the practice in the United Kingdom at the time.

EVIDENCE OF THE EXPERTS

[1] Professor Vallance – Written Evidence
"It is my opinion that in view of the earlier ambulatory readings, and the gradual increase in blood pressure during October and November, the interval between the clinic appointment on 29 November 1995, and January 24, 1996, was too long, and some attempt should have been made to have blood pressure measurements taken, and acted upon in the interim, within four weeks of 29 November. Mr Lowe's blood pressure was very significantly elevated on 4 January, 1996. As soon as this was known, some action should have been taken, ideally within 48 hours. Prompt control of his blood pressure at this stage, would have reduced the risk of a second bleed, so that on the balance of probabilities, the second bleed on 25 January would have been avoided. It is my opinion that failure to act upon this information about his blood pressure, falls below acceptable standards of care."

[2] Professor O'Grady – Oral Evidence

He said that his criticisms of Dr Pearson begin after 29 November. If the interval was as long as 8 weeks, there had to be some monitoring of the blood pressure. A home reading could be substituted, or a reading by a general practitioner, or by the 24-hour ambulatory reading. He said if that was done, it had to be done at some reasonable mid-period in the 8 weeks. As for the ambulatory tests, Professor O'Grady said that when the results of the ambulatory tests became available, they were extremely alarming, and they called for action, if not that day, then the next. If Dr Pearson did not see the results until 17 January, and did nothing for seven or eight days until 24 January, this was not proper. It was at this point in his evidence that Professor O'Grady made the point that hypertension is a fatal disease if untreated. The evidence of Professors Vallance and O'Grady was considered clear and uncompromising. They both thought that Dr Pearson had failed to comply with a proper standard of care.

[3] Dr Thomas – Oral Evidence

Dr Thomas stated that Dr Pearson wanted to get a 24-hour ambulatory blood pressure which was true. It was reasonable to build in a period of delay in order to complete the test. It was not unreasonable to set the next outpatient appointment 8 weeks later. It was reasonable, he thought, to order a 24-hour ambulatory blood pressure recording, and reasonable to allow time for that to happen. He stated that the claimant did not need to be seen by any medical practitioner for seven to eight weeks. On the other aspect of the claim, Dr Thomas said that he did not accept that after the ambulatory blood pressure recordings became known, it was so urgent as to require attention within 48 hours. He further stated that reviewing the patient within two weeks was reasonable.

[4] Professor Brown – Oral Evidence
Professor Brown agreed that the ambulatory blood pressure recordings showed an urgent, but not an emergency condition. He stated that a two-week wait was reasonable for a response to a risk of this order, that is to say, 2.5% per annum. He also expressed that his opinion was based on the risk in general for patients in the same position as Mr Lowe.

THE JUDGE'S CONCLUSIONS

"It appeared to me that both Dr Thomas and Professor Brown failed to make sufficient allowance for various special aspects of the claimant's condition, as described by Professors Vallance and O'Grady. There were a number of these. The first was that the claimant had not only a high blood pressure, but an uncontrolled one, it went up to high levels and then down irregularly and responded poorly to treatment. Secondly, there was a suspicion, voiced by Dr Pearson to his colleague, that the claimant may not have been fully compliant with the medication prescribed for him. There is in fact, no evidence in my judgment to justify a conclusion that at the material time, that is to say, 29 November onwards, the claimant was not fully compliant. Third, the claimant was a relatively young man to be suffering from this disorder. He had a wife and a dependent family. These are not medical considerations, they are social considerations of course, but they are considerations which a physician should, in my judgement, properly take into account in considering the general care of his patient.

Now it appears to me that both Dr Thomas and Professor Brown gave their evidence on as it were, general principles, and without taking into account any special; aspects of the claimant's condition. It seems to me that the claimant was not quite an ordinary patient. He was not a patient to whom the ordinary rules would apply without

further consideration. It is plain that Dr Pearson gave these factors no particular consideration, nor does it appear to me that in reading their opinions Dr Thomas or Professor Brown gave consideration to the claimant's personal characteristics which placed him in a category which required rather more care than the norm, rather than less. For the reasons which I have given earlier, I prefer the evidence of Professor Vallance and Professor O'Grady to that of Dr Thomas and Professor Brown where they are in conflict. And I accept, therefore, Professor O'Grady's evidence that the risk would have been reduced by at least 50% if the medication had been changed as late as early January. It follows from my findings of fact, that I find that Dr Pearson was negligent, and in breach of duty, in fixing an eight-week review period as from 29 November, and in failing to act on the ambulatory blood pressure readings earlier than 24 January. I find that both the first and second of those breaches were causative. Of the claimant's loss. I find, therefore, that the claimant succeeds on the issue of liability."
Source: Butterworths Medico-Legal Report (62, BMLR (2001) pp 69-83).

CASE THREE

CHESTER v AFSHAR

THE HOUSE OF LORDS

LORD BINGHAM OF CORNHILL; LORD STEYN;
LORD HOFFMANN, LORD HOPE OF CRAIGHEAD
AND LORD WALKER OF GESTINGTHORPE.

JULY – OCTOBER, 2004

Counsel for Claimant: Adrian Whitfield QC and Jacqueline
Perry.
Counsel for the Defendant: Martin Spencer QC and
Kristina Stern.

CASE SUMMARY

The claimant, Miss Chester, suffered from severe back pain
and was referred to the defendant who is an eminent
consultant neurosurgeon, who advised her to have surgery.
Three days later, the surgeon conducted the operation with
the patient's consent. Although the operation was properly
performed, it resulted in significant nerve damage, and left
the patient partially paralysed. Such damage was known to
be an inherent risk of the operation, in the region of 1-2%.
In subsequent proceedings for negligence, the patient
alleged that the surgeon had failed to advise her of that risk,
and that a breach of duty entitled her to damages. The judge
found that the surgeon had not informed the patient of the
risk before the operation; that he had been negligent in not
doing so, that if the patient had known of the risk, she
would not have consented to the operation at that time, and
that she would instead have sought a second or possibly a
third opinion before deciding what to do. It was on that

basis, that the judge concluded that the patient had established a causal link between the breach of duty and the injury, even though he made no finding. He gave judgment for the patient on the issue of liability, and his decision was affirmed by the Court of Appeal.

The surgeon appealed to the House of Lords, contending that, in order to establish causation in the case of a surgeon's failure to warn a patient of a significant risk of injury, the patient had to prove not only that she would not have consented to run the relevant risk then and there, but also that she would not at any time have consented to run the relevant risk.

In the Appeal to the House of Lords (Lord Bingham and Lord Hoffmann dissenting) it was stated that where, in breach of duty, a surgeon failed to warn a patient about a risk of injury inherent in an operation, and, as a result of that failure, the patient had the operation, and the risk materialised, she did not have to prove for the purpose of establishing causation, that she would never have had the operation at any time if properly warned. Rather, it was sufficient for her to prove that, if properly warned, she would not have consented to the operation which was in fact performed, and which resulted in the injury. Such a conclusion could not be based on 'conventional causation principles', because the risk was not created or increased by the failure to warn, and the chances of avoiding it were not lessened by that failure.

In such a case, however, justice required the normal approach to causation to be modified. The law which imposed the duty to warn on the doctor, had at its heart, the right of the patient to make an informed choice as to whether, and if so when, and by whom the operation would be performed. Patients were entitled to hold different views about these matters. For some, the choice might be easy, simply to agree or to decline the operation. For many, however, the choice would be a difficult one, requiring time to think, to take advice, and to weigh up the alternatives. The duty was owed as much to the patient who, if warned, would find the decision simple, and could give a clear answer to the doctor one way or another immediately, and to the patient who would find the decision difficult without a remedy, as the normal approach to causation would indicate. This would render the duty useless in the cases where it might be needed most. That would discriminate against those who could not honestly say that they would have decided the operation once and for all if they had been warned. That result was unacceptable. The function of the law was to enable rights to be vindicated and to provide remedies when the duties had been breached.

Unless that was done, the duty was a hollow one, stripped of all practical force and devoid of all content. It will have lost its ability to protect the patient and thus to fulfil the only purpose which brought it into existence. It followed that, on policy grounds, the test of causation was satisfied in the instant case. The injury was the product of the very risk that the patient should have been warned about when she gave her consent, and it could therefore be regarded as having been caused in the legal sense, by the breach of duty to warn. Accordingly, the appeal would be dismissed.

The defendant, Fari Afshar, appealed with permission of the Appeal Committee of the House of Lords, given on 18, November, 2002, from the order of the Court of Appeal (Hale, LJ, Sir Christopher Slade and Sir Denis Henry), on 27, May, 2002, dismissing his appeal from the order of Judge Robert Taylor, sitting as a judge of the High Court on 21 December, 2000, giving judgment for the claimant, Carole Gay Ogilvy Chester, for damages to be assessed in her proceeding for negligence against Mr Afshar. The facts of the case are set out in the opinions of the five Law Lords. Their Lordships took time for consideration and on 14, October, 2004, the following opinions were delivered.

COURT TRANSCRIPTS (EXTRACTS)

[1] LORD BINGHAM OF CORNHILL

"The central question in this appeal is whether the conventional approach to causation in negligence actions should be varied where the claim is based on a doctor's negligent failure to warn a patient of a small but unavoidable risk of surgery when, following surgery performed with due care and skill, such risk eventuates, but it is not shown that, if duly warned, the patient would not have undergone surgery with the same small but unavoidable risk of mishap. It is relevant to the outcome of the claim to decide whether duly warned, the patient probably would or probably would not have consented to undergo the surgery in question.

For some six years, beginning in 1988, the claimant Miss Chester, suffered repeated episodes of low back pain. She was treated by Dr Wright, a consultant rheumatologist, who administered epidural and sclerosant injections. An MRI scan in 1992 showed evidence of disc protrusions. In 1994, on the eve of a professional trip abroad, Miss Chester suffered another episode of pain and disability; she could hardly walk and had reduced control of her bladder.

Dr Wright gave another epidural injection and Miss Chester was able to make her trip, using a wheelchair at Heathrow. After the trip the pain returned. A further MRI scan revealed marked protrusion of discs into the spinal canal. After further conservative treatment which proved ineffective, Dr Wright referred Miss Chester to Mr Afshar, a distinguished consultant neurosurgeon with much experience of disc surgery, although Miss Chester was understandably reluctant to undergo surgery if this could be avoided.

On accepting Miss Chester as a patient, Mr Afshar

became subject to a legal as well as a professional duty to exercise reasonable care and skill in examining her, in assessing her case, and in advising on the need for surgery to alleviate the condition. If surgery was advised and accepted, he was bound to exercise reasonable care and skill in operating and supervising her post-operatively. Mr Ashar did examine Miss Chester, did advise and did undertake surgery. All these duties Mr Afshar duly performed.

Miss Chester contended at trial that Mr Afshar had performed the operation negligently. However, the judge at the trial rejected this complaint, and in the event, the Court of Appeal was not asked to rule on that question. However, Mr Afshar was subject to a further important duty to warn Miss Chester of a small (1%-2%) unavoidable risk that the proposed operation might lead to a seriously adverse result. This in medicine is called 'cauda equina' syndrome. The cauda equina is a bundle of nerve roots from the lumbar, sacral and coccygeal spinal nerves that descend almost vertically from the spinal cord until they reach their respective openings in the vertebral column.

The existence of such a duty is not in doubt. Nor is its rationale; to enable adult patients of sound mind to make for themselves, decisions intimately affecting their own lives and bodies. There was a conflict of evidence at trial on what was said by Mr Afshar about the risk of an adverse outcome. However, the judge resolved this conflict against him, holding that he had not given the warning which he should have given, and the Court of Appeal did not give him leave to challenge that conclusion. It must be accepted that Mr Afshar did not give Miss Chester the warning which he should have given of the small but unavoidable risk that surgery might not improve Miss Chester's condition but might affect it adversely. As it was, the surgery, although skilfully performed, led to her suffering the cauda equina syndrome.

Had the evidence entitled the judge to conclude and he had concluded, that Miss Chester if warned as she should have been, would probably not have agreed to surgery, she would on conventional principles, have been entitled to recover damages. The measure of damages would have reflected the difference between Miss Chester's condition following surgery, and the condition she would probably have been in without surgery, but there would have been no problem of causation. Had the warning been given, Miss Chester would have acted differently, and her additional injury would be directly attributable to the absence of warning. The same would be true if the evidence had entitled the judge to conclude, and if he had concluded, that Miss Chester, if properly warned as she should have been, could and would have minimised the risk of surgery by entrusting herself to a different surgeon, or undergoing a different form of surgery.

But the judge made none of these findings. He concluded that, if duly warned, Miss Chester would not have undergone surgery three days after her first consultation with Mr Afshar but would, very understandably, have wished to discuss the matter with others and explore other options. But he did not find that she would probably not have undergone the surgery or there was any way of minimising the small degree of risk in surgery. In the ordinary run of cases, satisfying the 'but for' test is a necessary condition of establishing causation. Here, in my opinion, it is not satisfied. Miss Chester has not established that; 'but for' the failure to warn, she would not have undergone surgery. The question arises whether Miss Chester should be entitled to recover even though she cannot show that the negligence proved against Mr Afshar, was a cause of her loss.

A claimant is entitled to be compensated for the damage which the negligence of another has caused him or her. A defendant is bound to compensate the claimant for the damage which his or her negligence has caused the claimant. But the corollaries are also true; a claimant is not entitled to be compensated, and a defendant is not bound to compensate the claimant for damages not caused by the negligence complained of. I do not for my part, think that the law should seek to reinforce that right by providing for the payment of potentially very large damages by a defendant whose violation of that right is not shown to have worsened the physical condition of the claimant. For those reasons, I would allow this appeal."

[2] LORD STEYN

"The facts of this case can be simplified. The claimant suffered from low back pain. A neurosurgeon advised her to undergo an elective lumber surgical procedure. The procedure entails a 1%-2% serious neurological damage arising from the operation. The claimant was entitled to be informed of this fact. In breach of the common law duty of care, the surgeon failed to inform the claimant of the risk. The claimant reluctantly agreed to the operation. Three days after her consultation with the surgeon, the claimant underwent the surgery. The claimant sustained serious neurological damage. This resulted in the very injury about which she should have been warned occurring. The surgeon had not been negligent in performing the operation; he did not increase the risks inherent in the surgery. On the other hand, if the claimant had been warned she would not have agreed to the operation. Instead, she would have sought further advice on alternatives. The judge found that if the claimant had been properly warned, the operation would not have taken place when it did, if at all.

The judge was unable to find whether if the claimant had been duly warned, she would with the benefit of further medical advice, have given or refused consent to surgery. What is clear is that she had agreed to surgery at a subsequent date, the risk attendant upon it would have been the same. It is therefore improbable that she would have sustained neurological damage. On these facts, the judge found that the claimant had established a causal link between the breach and the injury she had sustained, and held that the defendant was liable for damages. In a detailed and careful judgment, the Court of Appeal upheld the conclusion of the judge.

The legal context requires consideration of a number of other relevant factors. First, the nature of the correlative rights and duties of the patient and the surgeon, must be kept in mind. The starting point is that every individual of adult years and sound mind has a right to decide what may or may not be done with his or her body. Individuals have a right to make important medical decisions affecting their lives for themselves, they have the right to make decisions which doctors regard as ill-advised. Surgery performed without the informed consent of the patient is unlawful. The court is the final arbiter of what constitutes informed consent. Usually, informed consent will presuppose a general warning by the surgeon of a significant risk of the surgery. In the case before the House, a single cause of action is under consideration, the tort of negligence.

A surgeon owes a legal right to a patient to warn him or her in general terms of the possible serious risks involved in the procedure. A patient's right to an appropriate warning from a surgeon when faced with the surgery ought normatively be regarded as an important right which must be given effective protection whenever possible. It is a distinctive feature of this present case that 'but for' the surgeon's negligent failure to warn the claimant of the small risk of serious injury, the actual injury would not have occurred when it did, and the chance of it occurring on a subsequent occasion was very small. It could, therefore, be said that the breach of the surgeon resulted in the very injury about which the claimant was entitled to be warned.

I have come to the conclusion that, as a result of the surgeon's failure to warn the patient, she cannot be said to have given informed consent to the surgery in the full legal sense. Her right of autonomy and dignity can and ought to be vindicated by a narrower and modest departure from traditional causation principles. On a broader basis, I am glad to have arrived at the conclusion that the claimant is entitled in law to succeed."

[3] LORD HOFFMANN

"The purpose of a duty to warn someone against the risk involved in what he proposes to do, or allow to be done to him, is to give him 'the opportunity to avoid or reduce that risk'. If he would have been unable or unwilling to take that opportunity and the risk eventuates, the failure to warn has not caused the damage, it would have happened anyway. The burden is on a claimant to prove that the defendant's breach of duty caused him damage. Where the breach of duty is a failure to warn of a risk, he must prove that he would have taken the opportunity to avoid or reduce the risk. In the context of the present case, that means proving that she would not have had the operation. The judge made no finding that she would not have had the operation. He was not invited by the claimant to make such a finding. The claimant argued that as a matter of law, it was sufficient that she would not have had the operation at that time or by that surgeon, even though the evidence was that the risk could have been precisely the same if she had it at another time or by another surgeon. The judge found as a fact, that the risk would have been precisely the same whether it was done then or later or by that competent surgeon or by another. It follows that the claimant failed to prove that the defendant's breach of duty caused her loss. On ordinary principles of tort law, the defendant is not liable. I would allow the Appeal and dismiss the action."

[4] LORD HOPE OF CRAIGHEAD

"The appellant, Mr Fari Afsher, is an eminent consultant neurosurgeon. He carries on his practice both under the National Health Service and privately. The respondent, Miss Carole Chester, was formerly a working journalist specialising in travel writing. On 18 November 1994, she attended a consultation with Mr Afshar as a private patient in his consulting rooms in Harley Street. She had suffered for several years from back pain, and had been referred to him by another medical practitioner with a view to surgery. Three days later, on 21 November, 1994, Mr Afshar conducted an operation on Miss Chester's back, with her consent. It resulted in significant nerve damage and left her partially paralysed. Miss Chester's case that the operation was performed negligently was rejected by the High Court trial judge (Robert Taylor). He held that she failed to establish that Mr Afshar was in anyway negligent in his conduct of her surgery. However, Miss Chester also claimed that Mr Afshar failed to advise her of the risks inherent in the operation, and that this breach of duty entitled her to damages. The trial judge found that the injury which she had sustained during surgery, was caused by Mr Afshar's negligence in failing adequately to advise her of the risks of surgery, and that on this ground, she had established liability.

The Court of Appeal in 2002 dismissed Mr Afshar's appeal against this finding by the trial judge. The issue of law in the case rests upon two findings of fact by the trial judge. The first is his finding that Miss Chester was not told, pre-operatively of the risk of nerve damage possibly resulting in paralysis. Mr Afshar said that while he could not remember verbatim what he said to her, he thought that he spent a good deal of time spelling out what the risks were. But the trial judge was satisfied that she was not given adequate or proper advice about the risk of nerve damage possibly resulting in paralysis, and that despite her requests for information about such risks, she was given to understand in effect that there were none. He found that in this respect, Mr Afshar was negligent. The second was his finding that, if she had known of the actual risks of the proposed surgery, Miss Chester would not have consented to the operation taking place on 21 November, 1994, and that before deciding what to do, she would have sought a second or possibly a third opinion.

The question of law which arises from these findings is whether it was sufficient for Miss Chester to prove that, if properly warned, she would not have consented to the operation, which was in fact performed and which resulted in the injury, or whether it was necessary for her to prove also that she would never have had that operation. The issue is essentially one of causation. It is not disputed that the failure to warn could be said to have caused the injury if Miss Chester's position had been that she would never have undertaken the operation at all if that warning had been given. However, as the trial judge observed, it was one of the signs of her truthfulness that Miss Chester did not attempt to go that far, as she had never claimed that, if adequately advised of the risks, she would never at any time have consented to surgery. Can it then be said on these facts, that the test for causation is satisfied?

It was not in dispute that 'causa equina' damage was a known risk of the surgery which was performed by Mr Afshar who stated that the risk of such damage was about 0.9%. It was also common ground at the trial that it was Mr Afshar's duty in accordance with good medical practice, to warn Miss Chester of the risk of damage involved in the surgery., to which she was giving her consent, and its possible consequences, including the risk of paralysis. The Court of Appeal was asked to give permission to appeal against the judge's factual findings on the case as to whether she was told of these risks. The Court was of the opinion that the judge had given detailed and compelling reasons for preferring the claimant's account of her conversation with Mr Afshar. It held that there were no grounds that would justify interfering with his findings of facts.

The right to make a final decision and the duty of the doctor to inform the patient if the treatment may have special disadvantages or dangers, go hand in hand. In this case, there is no dispute that Mr Afshar owed a duty to Miss Chester to inform her of the risks that were inherent in the proposed surgery, including the risk of paralysis. The duty was owed to her so that she could make her own decision as to whether or not she should undergo the particular course of surgery which he proposed to carry out. That was the scope of the duty, the existence of which gave effect to her right to be informed before she consented to it. There were three possibilities. She might have agreed to go ahead with the operation despite the risks. Or she might have decided then and there not to have the operation, then or at any time in the future. Or she might have decided not to have the operation then, but to think the matter over and take further advice, leaving the possibility of having the operation open for the time being. The choice between these alternatives was for her to take and for her alone. The function of the law is to protect the patient's rights to choose. If it is to fulfil that function, it must ensure that the duty to inform is respected by the doctor.

The law which imposed the duty to warn on the doctor has at its heart, the right of the patient to make an informed choice, as to whether, and if so, when and by whom, to be operated on. Patients may have, and are entitled to have, different views about these matters. All sorts of factors may be at work here, the patient's hopes and fears, and personal circumstances, the nature of the condition that has to be treated, and, above all, the patient's own views about whether the risk is worth running for the benefits that may come if the operation is carried out. For some, the choice may be easy, simply to agree to or decline the operation. But for many the choice will be a difficult one, requiring time to think, to take advice and to weigh up the alternatives. The duty is owed as much to the patient who, if warned, would find the decision difficult as to the patient who would find it simple, and could give a clear answer to the doctor one way or the other immediately.

To leave the patient who would find the decision difficult without a remedy, as the normal approach to causation would indicate, would render the duty useless in the cases where it may be needed most. The function of the law is to enable rights to be vindicated and to provide remedies when duties have been breached. Unless this is done, the duty is a hollow one stripped of all practical force and devoid of all impact. It will have lost its ability to protect the patient and thus to fulfil the only purpose which brought it into existence. On policy ground, I would hold that the test of causation is satisfied in this case. The injury was intimately involved with the duty to warn. The duty was owed by the doctor who performed the surgery that Miss Chester consented to. It was the product of the very risk that she should have been warned about when she gave her consent.

I would hold that it can be regarded as having been caused, in the legal sense, by the breach of that duty. I would hold that justice requires that Miss Chester be afforded the remedy which she seeks, as the injury which she suffered at the hands of Mr Afshar was within the scope of the very risk which she should have been warned about, when he was obtaining her consent to the operation which resulted in that injury. I would dismiss the appeal."

[5] LORD WALKER OF GESTINGTHORPE

"The issue of 'causation' cannot be properly addressed without a clear understanding of the scope of the defendant's duty, in this case, the surgeon's duty to warn his patient of the risk, small though it was, of nerve damage occurring during lumbar surgery. The surgeon's duty to advise his patient (and in particular to warn of unavoidable risks of surgery) is a very important part of his professional duty. This duty to advise and warn his patient is closely connected with the need for the patient's consent to submit under anaesthesia, to invasive surgery which would, (in the absence of consent), be an assault.

The advice is the foundation of the consent. In this case, the surgeon failed to warn of the risk of the very calamity which occurred in the course of the operation which he performed three days later. As Lord Hope points out, of an honest claimant finding herself without a remedy in circumstances where the surgeon has failed in his professional duty, and the claimant has suffered injury directly within the scope and focus of that duty. I agree with Lord Steyn and Lord Hope that such a claimant ought not to be without a remedy. I would dismiss the appeal."

In this case, the House of Lords considered for the first time, whether the decision to postpone a proceeding has sufficient normative power to justify attributing casual responsibility in failure to warn cases. The House of Lords by a three to two minority, held that it did, and upheld the Court of Appeal's decision. Following this particular case, the law is now left with a relatively clear rule that it will be sufficient to establish causation in failure to warn cases, provided the patient would have at least, postponed the operation. If the autonomy argument is accepted, then the logical consequence of this is that the patient should also be able to recover damages if the undisclosed risk materialises, even where disclosure would not have altered the patient's decision.

Source: Butterworths Medico-Legal Reports, 81 BMLR (2004) pp 1-32.

EPILOGUE

"The crucial question is that of determining the extent to which medical decisions should be the object of legal scrutiny and control. At one extreme, there are those who hold that the medical profession should be left to regulate itself, and that it alone should decide what is acceptable conduct. According to this view, intervention by the law is too blunt a way of tackling the delicate ethical dilemmas which doctors have to face. The individual guided by personal experience and by prevailing public and professional standards, must confront and resolve the day-to-day ethical issues of medical practice. There is no doubt that the intrusion of the law into the doctor/patient relationship, essential as it may be in some instances, leads to a subtle but important change in the nature of the relationship. Trust and respect are more likely to flourish in one which is governed by morality rather than by legal rules, and the injection of formality, and excessive caution between doctor and patient cannot be in the patients' interest if it means that each sees the other as a potential adversary.

Where then, does the doctor stand today in relation to society? To some extent, and perhaps increasingly, he is a servant of the public, a public which is, moreover, widely – though not always well-informed on medical matters. The competent patients' inalienable rights to understand his treatment and to accept or refuse it are now well established, and society is conditioned to distrust professional paternalism. It is, moreover, in many ways, extraordinary that the provision of a national health service which one would have thought should above all other services, be free of bias, has, in recent years, become perhaps the main political issue that determines the voters' intentions in the United Kingdom. As a result, more and more extravagant claims and more significantly, promises, are made with little regard for the fallibility and limitations of those who must implement them.

Unless humanity of both health carers and patients is appreciated by both sides and is not exploited in the political arena, the resulting disappointment on both sides, may well lead to a relationship of conflict or of mutual suspicion, which is in the interests of neither doctor nor patient. What is needed is one of mutual understanding, in which doctors acknowledge the interests of patients, and patients, for their part, reciprocate this respect while appreciating the pressures, both physical and mental, under which a health carer must work."

Source: JK Mason, RA McCall Smith, and GT Laurie - "Law and Medical Ethics" (6th Edition) (Butterworths, London, 2002, pp 22-25).

BIBLIOGRAPHY AND REFERENCES

Publications

Brazier, M, *Medicine, Patients and the Law* (3rd edition) (Penguin Books, 2003).

Brazier, M & Murphy, J (Eds), *Street on Torts* (10th Edit, Butterworths, London, 1999).

Byrne, P (Ed), *Medicine in Contemporary Society* (King's Fund Institute, Oxford, 1987).

Danzan, M, *Medical Malpractice* (Harvard University Press, Cambridge, Mass, 1985).

Davies, M, *Textbook on Medical Law* (2nd Edit, Oxford University Press, 1998).

Dworkin, G, *The Theory and Practice of Autonomy* (Cambridge University Press, New York,1988).

Freeman, MDA, (Ed), *Medicine, Ethics and Law* (Stevens, London, 1988).

Gert, B & Culver, CM, *Philosophy in Medicine* (Oxford University Press, New York, 1982).

Hacking, I, *The Emergence of Probability* (Cambridge University Press, 1975).

Harris, C, Dingwall, R & Fenn, P, *Medical Negligence, Compensation and Accountability* (King's Fund Institute, Oxford, 1988).

Hill, TE, *Autonomy and Self-Respect* (Cambridge University Press, 1991).

Kennedy, I & Grubb, A, *Medical Law, Text and Materials* (Butterworths, London. 2000).

Lewis, R, *Structured Settlements* (Sweet and Maxwell, London, 1996).

Mason, JK Smith, McCall, A & Laurie, GT, *Law, and Medical Ethics* (6th Edit, Butterworths, London, 1999).

Merry, A & Smith, McCall A, *Errors, Medicine and the Law* (Cambridge University Press, 2003).
Teff, H, *Reasonable Care* (Oxford: Clarendon Press, 1994).

ARTICLES

Medical Law Review (Med LR)
I Kennedy, 'The Patient on the Clapham Omnibus' (1984. 47, Med LR 454)
A McCall Smith, 'Criminal Negligence and the Incompetent Doctor' (1993: 1, Med LR 336).
MA Jones, 'Informed Consent and Other Fairy Stories' (1999, Med LR 103).
J Burrows, 'Telling Tales and Savings Lives: Whistleblowing – The Role of Professional Colleagues in Protecting Patients from Dangerous Doctors' (2001, 9, Med LR103).
A Grubb, 'Clinical Negligence, Informed Consent and Causation' (2002 10, Med LR 322)'
Stauch M, 'Taking the Consequences for Failing to Warn of Medical Risks', (2004, 63 Med LR, 261.)
Nottingham Law Journal (NLJ).
A Maclean, 'Risk, Consent and Responsibility for Outcomes' (NLJ Vol 14 (1) 2005 pp57-65).
M Stauch, 'Causation and Confusion in Respect of Medical Non-Disclosure' (NLJ, Vol 14 (1), 2005, pp 66-72)

British Medical Journal (BMJ)
R Smith, 'Doctors, Unethical Treatment and Turning a Blind Eye' (1989 298-1125).
B Capstick, P Edwards & Mason, 'Compensation for Medical Accidents' (1991 302-230).
JA Devereux, D Jones & DI Dickenson 'Can Children Withhold Consent to Treatment?' (1993, 306-1459).
B Hurwitz, 'Clinical Guidelines and the Law' (1993) 311-1517).

J Mitchell, 'A Fundamental Problem of Consent' (1995, 340, 43).
J Harris, 'The Injustice of Compensation for Victims of Medical Accidents' (1997, 314, 182).
C Dyer, 'Bristol Doctors Found Guilty of Serious Professional Misconduct' (1998, 316, 1924).
C Dyer, 'GPs Face Escalating Litigation' (1999, 318, 830).
RE Ferner, 'Medication Errors that have led to Manslaughter Charges' (2000, 321, 1212).
S Dewer & B Finlayson, 'Dealing with Poor Clinical Performance' (2001, 322-66).
KG Alberti, 'Medical Errors: A Common Problem' (2001, 322, 501).
DP Gray, 'De- Professionalising Doctors' (2002, 324, 627).
K Walshe, 'The Rise of Regulation in the NHS' (2002, 324, 967).

Government Inquiries and Reports

Access to Justice Final Report to the Lord Chancellor on the Civil Justice System in England and Wales (The Woolf Report) (HMSO, London, 1996).
Report of the Public Inquiry into Children's Heart Surgery at Bristol Royal Infirmary: 1984-1995).
(Cmnd 5207-2001) (www.bristol-inquiry.org.uk).
The Royal Liverpool Children's Inquiry Report (HC 12, 2001) (www. rlc-inquiry.org.uk).
Independent Inquiry into care provided by Mid-Staffordshire NHS Foundation Trust. January 2005 to March, 2009. Report - Robert Francis QC (Department of Health, London, 2010).
Royal Commission on Civil Liability and Compensation for Personal Injury Report (The Pearson Report) (Cmnd 7054, HMSO, London, 1978).

TABLE OF CASES

Barnett v Chelsea and Kensington Hospital Management Committee (1969), 1 QB 428.
Blyth v Birmingham Waterworks Co (1856), 11- Exch. 781.
Bolitho v City and Hackney Health Authority (1997), 4 All ER, 771 (HL).
Bolam v Friern Hospital Management Committee (1957), 2 All ER 118.
Cassidy v Ministry of Health, (1951), 2 KB 343. 1 All ER, 574, CA.
Chester v Afshar (2004). HL. 81, BMLR.
Crawford v Board of Governors of Charing Cross Hospital, The Times, 8, December, (1953).
Defreitas v O' Brien, (1995) AC 562.
Donaghue v Stevenson, (1932) AC. 562.
Dunning v Liverpool Hospitals' Board of Governors, (1973). 2 All ER. 454.
Glass v Cambridge Health Authority (1995), 6 Med LR, 91.
Hotson v East Berkshire Health Authority, (1987), 2 All ER.909, HL.
Hunter v Hanley, (1955) SC 200.
Kelly v Metropolitan Rly (1895), 1 QB, 944.
Lewis v Carmarthenshire County Council, (1953), 1 All ER. 1025.
Lowe v Havering Hospitals NHS Trust, (2001), QBD, 62. BMLR.
Ludlow v Swindon Health Authority, (1989), 1 Med L.R. 104.
Mahon v Osborne, (1939), 2 KB, 4.
N v UK Medical Research Council (1996), BMLR 83.
Naylor v Preston Area Health Authority, (1987), 2 All ER, 353.
Roe v Ministry of Health, (1954), 2 QB, 66.
Sidaway v Board of Governors of the Bethlehem Royal Hospital and the Maudsley Hospital (1984), 1 All ER, 643.

Whitehouse v Jordan, (1981) 1 All ER. 267.
Williamson v East London and City Health Authority, (1997), 41, BMLR, 85.
Wilster v Essex Area Health Authority, (1987), QB 730, 3 All ER, 801.
R v Bateman, (1925), 94, 1 JKB, 791.
R v Adomako, (1995), 1 AC.
Re T (adult: refusal of medical treatment), (1992), CA, BMLR,9.

Dr David Holding

Words Are Life's Best Selling Title

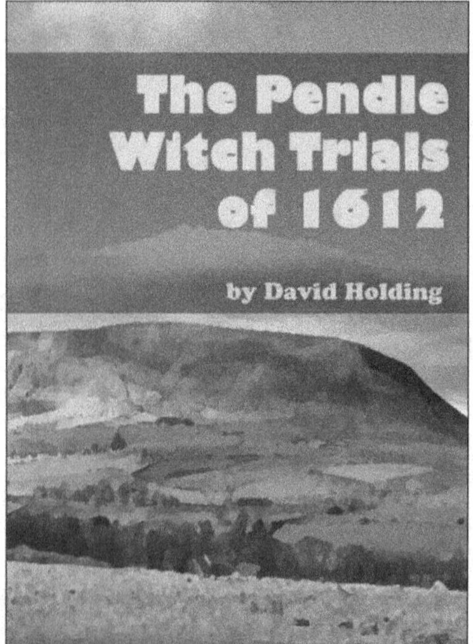

Sold world-wide to libraries, educational establishments and individuals, this is *"The Pendle Witch Trials of 1612"*.

What it doesn't do...

Sensationalise the historic trials and associated events.

Fictionalise the already-fascinating characters involved.

Romanticise or demonise the women accused of witchcraft— or their families.

What it does...

It provides an accurate account and overview of the court proceedings of 1612, and leaves the reader to make their own decision regarding the truth behind the infamous trials.

Currently available on Amazon

Kindle £3.50 and Paperback £5.50

ISBN: 9781797806679

www.wordarelife.co.uk

wordsarelife@mail.com

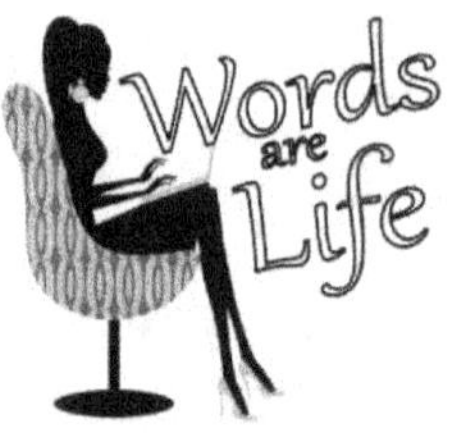

www.ingramcontent.com/pod-product-compliance
Lightning Source LLC
Chambersburg PA
CBHW050731260726
48661CB00001B/170